The LONGEVITY KITCHEN

Food as the First Prescription

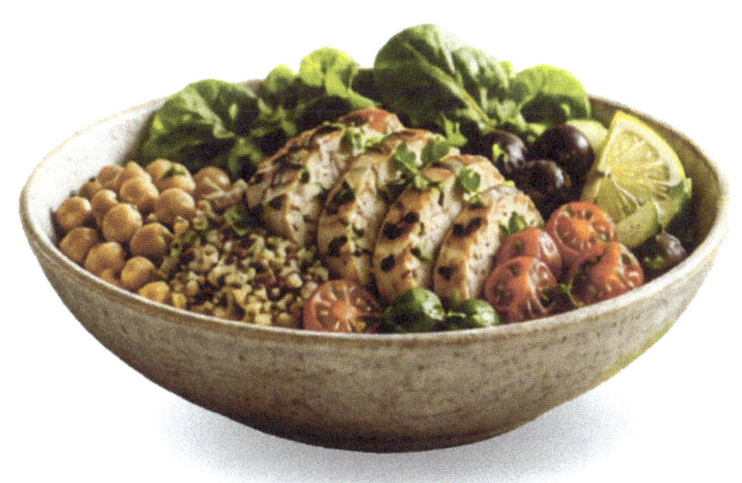

Written by

DR. DANIELA T. RIZZO, M.D.

The Longevity Kitchen

Medical Disclaimer:

This book is intended as a reference volume only, not as a medical manual. The information given here is designed to help you make informed decisions about your health. It is not intended as a substitute for any treatment that your doctor may have prescribed. If you suspect that you have a medical problem, we urge you to seek competent medical help.

The author and publisher specifically disclaim all responsibility for any liability, loss, or risk, personal or otherwise, that is incurred consequently, directly or indirectly, of the use and application of any of the contents of this book.

Mention of specific companies, organizations, or authorities in this book does not imply endorsement by the author or publisher, nor does mention of specific companies, organizations, or authorities imply that they endorse this book, its author, or the publisher.

Internet addresses and other contact information given in this book were accurate at the time of publication.

ISBN: 979-8-9954179-3-4

Published by: Rizzo Health Press
100 Park Ave., 16th Floor, New York, NY 10017

First Edition

10 9 8 7 6 5 4 3 2 1

Printed in the United States of America

For more information, visit:
drdanielarizzomd.com
Email: danielarizzomd@gmail.com

Bulk Purchase Information:

Personalized discounts are available on quantity purchases by corporations, associations, and others. For details, contact the publisher.

Nutrition/Medical Credentials Statement:

Dr. Daniela Rizzo is a board-certified physician and psychiatrist. The nutritional guidance in this book is based on peer-reviewed scientific literature and clinical experience. Individual results may vary. Always consult with your healthcare provider before making significant dietary changes, especially if you have existing medical conditions or take medications.

Recipe Testing Statement:

All recipes in this book have been tested for accuracy and palatability. Nutritional information is approximate and calculated using standard nutrition databases.

Epigraph

"Let food be thy medicine and medicine be thy food."

— Hippocrates

"The doctor of the future will give no medicine but will instruct his patients in care of the human frame, in diet, and in the cause and prevention of disease."

— Thomas Edison

"One cannot think well, love well, sleep well, if one has not dined well."

— Virginia Woolf

"To eat is a necessity, but to eat intelligently is an art."

— François de La Rochefoucauld

"The food you eat can be either the safest and most powerful form of medicine or the slowest form of poison."

— Ann Wigmore

Table of Contents

Dedication

For everyone who has ever been told a chronic disease is "just genetics." For those who refuse to accept that decline is inevitable. And for the next generation, who deserve to inherit better health than we did.

For my family in Brazil, whose struggles taught me that prevention is love.

For my husband, who proved that skeptics could become believers—and that it is never too late to choose health.

And for every patient who has ever sat across from me and asked, "Is there another way?"

There is. This book is that way.

Author's Note:
How To Use The Book

This Book Is Your Doctor's Appointment, Nutrition Consult, and Cooking Class—All in One

I designed The Longevity Kitchen to work the way medicine should: personalized, practical, and proven.

You do not need to read this book cover to cover (though you can). Instead, start where you are:

If You Are Facing A Health Crisis:

- Heart disease or high blood pressure? → Chapter 2: Prevention Before Prescription
- Type 2 diabetes or prediabetes? → Chapter 2 + 30-Day Plan in Chapter 6
- Cancer diagnosis or survivor? → Chapter 3: Cancer & Nutrition section
- Depression, anxiety, ADHD, or trauma? → Chapter 3: Mental Health sections

If You Want to Optimize Health:

- Curious about longevity science? → Chapter 4: Telomeres, NAD+, Fasting
- Athletic or high-performance goals? → Chapter 5: Peak Performance
- Just want to feel better? → Chapter 6: The 30-Day Roadmap

If You Are Ready To COOK:

- Jump straight to Chapter 7 for 26 tested recipes organized by meal type and health goal.

How the Science Works:

Every claim in this book is backed by peer-reviewed research. You will find citations throughout, with full references in the back matter. I am a physician and psychiatrist—I don't guess. I follow evidence.

A Note on Personalization:

This book provides general guidance based on population-level research. Always consult your physician before making significant dietary changes, especially if you:

- Take medications (food can interact)
- Have chronic conditions (diabetes, kidney disease, etc.)
- Are pregnant or breastfeeding
- Have a history of eating disorders

What You Won't Find Here:

- Miracle cures or quick fixes
- Expensive supplements as requirements
- Restriction or deprivation
- Judgment about where you're starting from

What You Will Find:

- Research-backed nutrition that works with (not against) modern medicine
- Real patient stories that prove change is possible
- Practical recipes designed for real kitchens and busy lives
- A roadmap you can start today, regardless of budget or cooking skills

My Promise to You:

If you commit to the principles in this book for 30 days, you will feel different. Your body will respond. Your numbers will improve. Your energy will return.

This is not theory. This is biology.

Let's begin.

About The Author

Dr. Daniela T. Rizzo, M.D.

Physician | Psychiatrist | Living Proof That Food Changes Everything

Dr. Daniela Rizzo is not your typical doctor.

In her psychiatric practice, Dr. Rizzo sees the pattern daily: patients on antidepressants who still feel flat, patients on mood stabilizers who still struggle, patients on stimulants who still can't focus.

When she asks about their diet, the answer is often the same: processed foods, irregular meals, lots of sugar, almost no vegetables.

She's watched hundreds of patients transform when nutrition partners with medication:

- Depression lifts more fully
- Anxiety calms more deeply
- ADHD becomes manageable
- Bipolar disorder stabilizes
- Trauma survivors reclaim resilience

Medication is not the enemy. Neither is food. They are partners.

The Philosophy

Dr. Rizzo's approach is simple but revolutionary:

Food is not alternative medicine. Food is foundational medicine.

Without it, even the most advanced medications fight uphill battles. With it, medications, therapies, and surgeries gain allies instead of enemies.

She believes that:

- 80% of chronic disease is preventable through lifestyle
- Most people don't need more willpower—they need better information
- Healthy eating doesn't mean bland, boring, or expensive
- Change is possible at any age, any starting point, any budget

The Mission

Dr. Rizzo wrote The Longevity Kitchen because she's tired of:

- Watching people suffer from preventable diseases
- Seeing patients on five medications when food could reduce them to two
- Hearing "I wish I'd known this sooner" from people facing heart disease, diabetes, cancer, and depression
- A healthcare system that waits for crisis instead of investing in prevention

Most of all, she's tired of people believing they are powerless.

The Proof

Dr. Rizzo doesn't just preach this philosophy—she lives it:

- Gave up sugar at 14 and never went back
- Maintained Mediterranean-style eating through medical school, residency, and decades of practice
- Overcame ADHD through the combination of medication and nutrition
- Helped her husband reverse hypertension in 90 days
- Guided hundreds of patients to diabetes remission, depression recovery, and cardiovascular improvement

If she can do it—and her skeptical husband can do it—anyone can.

The Credentials

- MD from medical school in São Paulo, Brazil
- Psychiatry Residency and US medical licensure
- 20+ years of clinical practice integrating nutrition with mental and physical health
- Board-certified physician and psychiatrist
- Researcher in nutritional psychiatry

Dr. Rizzo lives with her family and continues to practice integrative psychiatry. She still eats the way she did at fourteen—not because it's a diet, but because it's who she is.

The Longevity Kitchen is one of two books she is currently publishing, and it is written for every patient who ever asked, "Is there another way?"

Praise for The Longevity Kitchen

"Dr. Rizzo has written the book I wish I could give every patient. Clear, compassionate, and backed by rigorous science, The Longevity Kitchen shows that food is not just fuel—it's medicine. This book will change lives."

— Robin Khan, RN

"As a psychiatrist, I've long known that nutrition affects mental health, but few books explain the connection as clearly as this one. Dr. Rizzo bridges the gap between psychiatry and nutrition with wisdom, research, and real patient stories. Essential reading."

— Jacob M. Appel, MD, JD, MPhil, Author of ***Who Says You're Dead?*** and ***Phoning Home***, Mount Sinai School of Medicine, Bioethics & Psychiatry

"Finally, a book that doesn't just tell you what to eat—it shows you why it matters and how to actually do it. Dr. Rizzo's personal journey and patient transformations prove that sustainable change is possible. Inspiring and practical."

—Samuel Dang, MS, RDN, CDN

"This is the prevention manual our healthcare system desperately needs. Dr. Rizzo demonstrates with clarity and compassion that most chronic diseases are not inevitable—they are choices we make three times a day. Powerful and hopeful."

—Anthony Bracco

"From telomeres to neurotransmitters, from Blue Zones to cutting-edge longevity science, The Longevity Kitchen translates complex research into actionable wisdom. Dr. Rizzo proves that the future of medicine is already in our kitchens."

—Dr. Margaret Saide

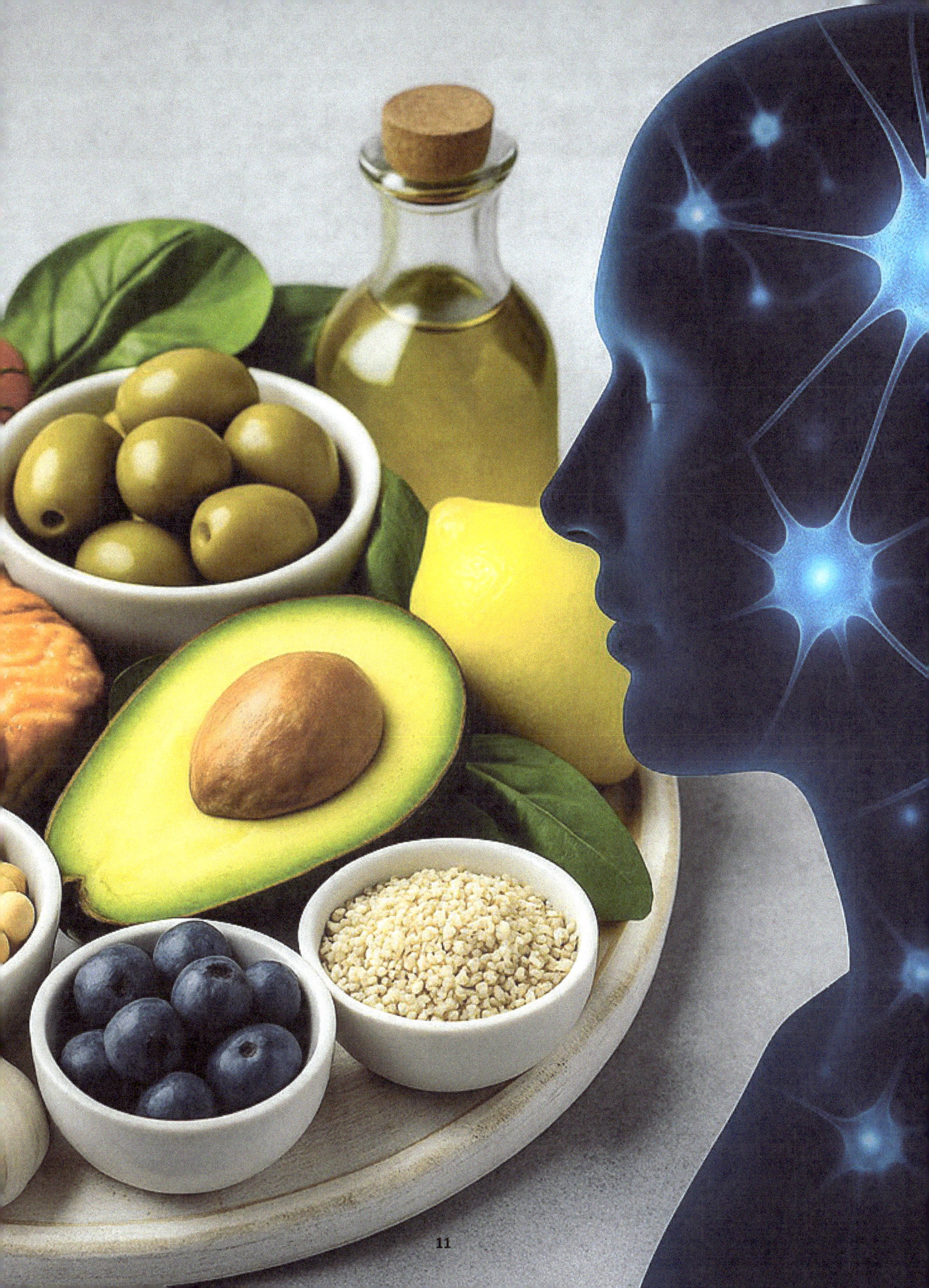

Introduction

My Journey from Sugar to Science

I was fourteen when I decided to give up sugar.

Not because the doctor told me to. Not because I was overweight or sick. But because I read something that changed everything: sugar ages the body. It accelerates disease. It shortens life.

At fourteen, most teenagers think about school dances, friendships, and weekend plans. I was thinking about longevity.

Growing up in Brazil, I watched family members suffer strokes, heart attacks, and hypertension. I saw relatives deteriorate from preventable diseases while continuing the very habits that made them sick. They did not know better. Or they knew but did not believe food could matter that much.

I believed food could be the difference.

So, I made a choice. I eliminated refined sugar from my diet. I started eating vegetables at every meal. I chose whole grains over white bread, water over soda, and fruit over candy. My friends thought I was extreme. My family thought I was obsessed.

But I was neither extreme nor obsessed. I was intentional.

That decision at fourteen set the course for my entire life. Through medical school in São Paulo, through psychiatry residency, through the grueling process of becoming a licensed physician in the United States—I never wavered. While classmates survived caffeine and fast food, I packed lunches of beans, vegetables, and olive oil. While colleagues grabbed vending machine snacks during overnight shifts, I carried almonds and fruit.

People asked why I cared so much. The answer was simple: I refused to accept my family's fate as my own.

The Challenge That Nearly Broke Me

But intention alone isn't always enough.

During my final step of medical licensure in the United States, I faced the hardest challenge of my life. I had ADHD—undiagnosed for years, unmedicated, unmanaged. The exam required sustained focus for hours. My mind couldn't hold still that long.

I failed. Then I failed again. And again. Five times total.

Each failure was devastating. Without passing this exam, I could not practice medicine in the United States. Everything I had worked for—medical school, residency, decades of discipline—meant nothing if I couldn't pass this test.

On my sixth attempt, I finally sought comprehensive help. I started ADHD medication. But medication alone wasn't enough. I restructured my entire life around focus:

- High-protein breakfasts to stabilize dopamine
- Omega-3 supplementation to support brain function.
- No sugar to prevent glucose crashes.
- Consistent hydration because even mild dehydration worsens attention.
- Daily exercise to improve executive function.
- Structured sleep to allow my brain to consolidate learning.

The medication opened the door. Nutrition walked me through it.

On exam day, for the first time in six attempts, my mind stayed present. I could read questions once and comprehend them. Time management held. Focus sustained.

I passed.

The Husband Who Proved Me Right

Years later, I married a man who loved me but didn't share my passion for nutrition. He ate what he wanted. He didn't exercise regularly. He thought my way of eating was "too strict."

Then, at age forty-five, his blood pressure spiked to 180/95. Dangerous.

Pre-stroke territory.

His doctor prescribed medication. I made a different offer: "Give me three months. Change your diet. Move your body. If it doesn't work, take the medication."

He agreed—reluctantly.

Within three months, his blood pressure normalized. No medication. Just beans, vegetables, olive oil, fish, walking, and sleep.

He became my most powerful case study. Because if he could change—a skeptic who resisted for years—then anyone can.

What I've Learned as a Psychiatrist

In my psychiatric practice, I see the same pattern repeat: patients on antidepressants who still feel flat, patients on mood stabilizers who still struggle, patients on stimulants who still can't focus.

Medication helps. But when I ask about their diet, the answer is often the same: processed foods, irregular meals, lots of sugar, almost no vegetables.

Their medications are trying to work in a body starved of the nutrients needed to make neurotransmitters, regulate inflammation, and support brain function. It's like trying to drive a car with no oil in the engine. The engine might run—but not for long, and not well.

When patients combine medication with anti-inflammatory eating, omega-3s, stable blood sugar, and regular movement, everything changes. Depression lifts more fully. Anxiety calms more deeply. ADHD becomes manageable. Bipolar disorder stabilizes.

Medication is not the enemy. Neither is food. They are partners. And too often, we ignore the most powerful partner of all.

Why I Wrote This Book

I wrote this book because I'm tired of watching people suffer from preventable diseases.

I'm tired of seeing patients on five medications when food could reduce them to two.

I'm tired of hearing "I wish I'd known this sooner" from people facing heart disease, diabetes, cancer, and depression.

I'm tired of a healthcare system that waits for a crisis instead of investing in prevention.

Most of all, I'm tired of people believing they are powerless.

You are not powerless.

You can lower your risk of heart disease by 30%.

You can cut your risk of type 2 diabetes in half.

You can triple your chance of depression remission.

You can protect your brain, strengthen your bones, support your gut, and extend your life—not someday with a miracle drug, but today, with what you put on your plate.

This book is for the fourteen-year-old who wants to take control before disease strikes.

It's for the forty-five-year-old whose blood pressure just spiked.

It's for the patient who has been on antidepressants for years but still doesn't feel quite right.

It's for parents who want to model health for their children.

It's for the skeptic who thinks "healthy eating" means bland, boring deprivation.

It's for anyone who's ever thought: "There has to be a better way." There is. And it starts in your kitchen.

What You'll Find in These Pages

This book is organized into 7 Chapters:

Chapter 1 - Food as the First Prescription

Chapter 2 - Prevention before Prescription

Chapter 3 - Healing Chronic Illness & Mental Health

Chapter 4 - The Science of Longevity

Chapter 5 - Peak Performance

Chapter 6 - The Roadmap to Regeneration

Chapter 7 - Recipes for Life

You'll meet patients whose lives transformed:

- Lisa, who reversed type 2 diabetes and came off insulin
- Michael, who lifted his depression when food partnered with medication
- Sofia, who has stayed cancer-free for 10 years through cruciferous vegetables and movement
- My husband, who normalized his blood pressure in three months without medication

...and many others whose stories prove that change is possible

You'll learn the science: telomeres that lengthen, mitochondria that regenerate, NAD+ that restores, inflammation that calms, neurotransmitters that balance.

And you'll discover that the food you need isn't exotic, expensive, or complicated. It's beans, vegetables, olive oil, fish, nuts, whole grains, and berries. The same foods humans have thrived on for millennia.

My Promise to You

I will not sugarcoat the truth: changing your diet requires effort. Cooking takes time. Breaking old habits is hard.

But I also promise you this:

You will feel better. More energy, clearer thinking, deeper sleep, and steadier mood.

Your numbers will improve. Lower cholesterol, better blood pressure, and stable blood sugar.

Your risk will drop. For heart disease, diabetes, cancer, and dementia.

And you will reclaim power over your health that you didn't know you had.

I gave up sugar at fourteen because I refused my family's fate.

I fought through ADHD because I believed food and focus could work together.

I watched my husband reverse hypertension because he finally chose change.

I've seen patients overcome diabetes, depression, and chronic disease—one meal at a time.

If we can do it, you can too.

Your kitchen is your pharmacy.

Your recipes are your prescriptions.

Your future begins now.

Welcome to The Longevity Kitchen.

Dr. Daniela T. Rizzo, M.D.

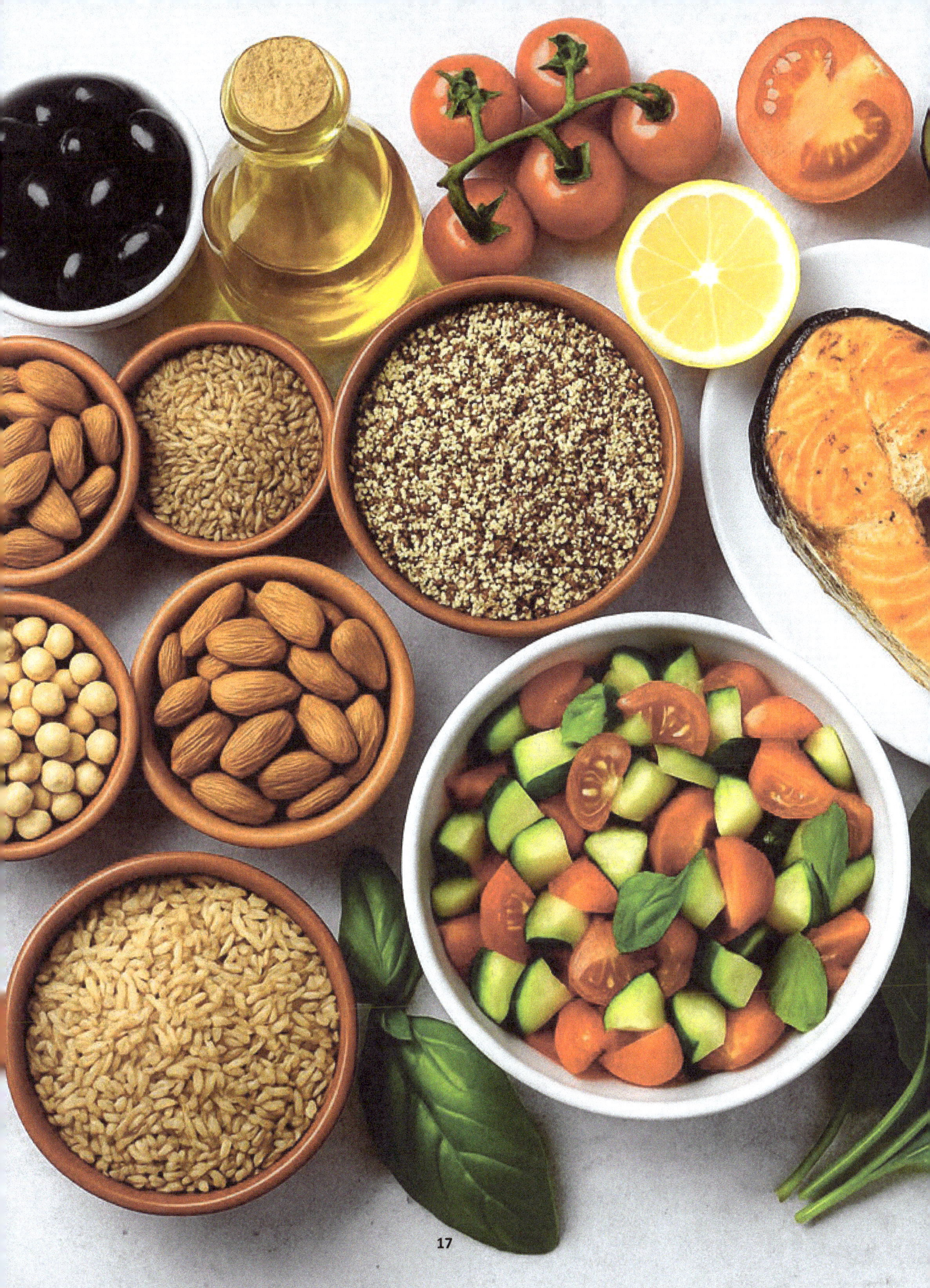

CHAPTER 1
Food as the First Prescription

A Life Defined by Choices

Every life is shaped by a series of quiet decisions.

Some choices feel small in the moment — what to eat, how to sleep, whether to exercise, whether to ignore or listen to the signals of the body. Yet over time these daily decisions accumulate, shaping the trajectory of health, longevity, and vitality.

When I chose to give up sugar at fourteen, I did not fully understand the biological consequences of that decision. I simply sensed that food had power — power to nourish the body or slowly undermine it. Years later, after medical school and clinical practice, science confirmed what intuition had whispered early on: food is not merely fuel. It is information.

Every meal sends signals to the body. Some calm inflammation and repair tissues. Others quietly accelerate disease.

This chapter explores why food became my first prescription, and why it should be the first prescription for anyone seeking a longer, healthier life.

It is a blueprint I wish every patient, every student, and every family member had received before the first pill was written. It's not an argument against medication—it's the foundation that makes medication work better.

Food does not only prevent disease. It repairs, regenerates, steadies the brain, and slows the cellular clock of aging.

SECTION 1: WHAT THE EVIDENCE SHOWS

The Mediterranean Pattern: Fewer Heart Attacks and Strokes

In a landmark trial published in the New England Journal of Medicine (2013), thousands of adults at high cardiovascular risk were assigned to one of three diets:

1. Mediterranean with extra virgin olive oil
2. Mediterranean with mixed nuts
3. Low-fat control

The investigators halted the study early because the benefit was too strong to ignore: 30% reduction in major cardiovascular events for the Mediterranean groups.

That is not a marginal effect—that is the kind of result we celebrate when it comes from a new drug. The difference here? Cost and side effects. The Mediterranean diet is accessible, and its side effects include better skin, better mood, and meals you want to eat again tomorrow.

Plant-Rich Eating: The Brain and Mood

Across pooled studies and controlled trials, people who eat plants, legumes, fish, whole grains, nuts, and olive oil have:

- Lower rates of depression and anxiety
- Better cognitive function into older age
- More stable energy and attention

The mechanisms are clear:

- Fiber feeds gut microbes that produce short-chain fatty acids, which calm inflammation
- Polyphenols protect neurons from oxidative stress
- Omega-3 fatty acids improve membrane fluidity and neurotransmitter signaling
- Steady glucose stabilizes energy and attention

When patients come to me with mood disorders, I discuss therapy and medication—but I also discuss magnesium, omega-3s, fermented foods, and breakfasts that contain protein rather than sugar.

Blue Zones: Long Lives Built in Kitchens

- In Okinawa, Sardinia, Ikaria, Nicoya, and Loma Linda, people live longer and better: fewer chronic diseases, more centenarians, more independent years.
- Their kitchens explain as much as their genetics:
- Beans most days

- Vegetables prepared simply
- Whole grains, nuts, seeds
- Olive oil as primary fat
- Extraordinarily little processed food
- Modest portions of fish
- Minimal red meat
- Alcohol, if at all, in negligible amounts with meals and community

Processed Foods: Faster Aging

On the opposite end, ultra-processed foods accelerate aging at multiple levels:

- Blood sugar spikes trigger glycation, stiffening collagen and deepening wrinkles
- Refined oils and additives amplify inflammation
- Repeated glucose-insulin surges exhaust metabolic flexibility
- Multiple cohorts show association between processed food intake and earlier death

None of this is abstract if you've watched a parent or sibling struggle. It's specific. It's day by day. It's what sits on a pantry shelf.

SECTION 2: FOUR LIVES CHANGED

CASE STUDY: Maria's Hypertension Reversal

Background: Maria, fifty-six, sat in her doctor's office with blood pressure reading 160/100 despite three medications. She was tired of swollen ankles, afternoon headaches, and sleep that never refreshed. Her diet reflected a life of convenience: white rolls with sweet coffee for breakfast, quick dinners of jarred sauces and salty foods, vegetables as decoration rather than substance.

The Challenge: Despite medications, her pressure remained dangerously high. Her family history mirrored mine—strokes, cholesterol, blame assigned to fate. She felt powerless.

The Intervention: We didn't start with perfection. We started with pantry. Together we removed crackers, cookies, instant noodles, and sugar-sweetened drinks. We replaced them with:

- Beans, olive oil, tomatoes, onions, garlic
- Barley, oats, walnuts
- Oranges, apples, frozen berries

Her meal structure:

- Breakfast rotation: Oatmeal with walnuts and blueberries (3 days), eggs with greens and whole grain toast (2 days), yogurt with chia seeds and fruit (weekends)
- Lunch: Lentil or bean-based soup with olive oil and vegetables
- Dinner template: Protein the size of her palm, generous vegetables, whole grain or potato, olive oil

The Results

- **Week 2:** Rings fit more easily in the morning
- **Month 2:** Blood pressure 138/87
- **Month 3: L**ost 5kg, blood pressure 130/82, no headaches in weeks
- **Month 6:** Average home readings 120/80, medications reduced, improved triglycerides and glucose

The Science: Maria's recovery reflects a study in Hypertension (2017): plant-rich diets reduce blood pressure as effectively as first-line medications. JAMA (2019) confirmed Mediterranean-style eating lowers blood pressure and cardiovascular events.

The Lesson: Maria didn't join a boot camp or count every calorie. She stocked food that loves her blood vessels—beans and greens, olive oil and nuts, whole grains that steady glucose, fruit that satisfies without the crash. Her story is common and powerful because it's achievable. "It feels like a different life," she said, "one that someone like me could live."

CASE STUDY: David's Depression Lifted

Background: David, thirty-two, described his life as gray. Antidepressants for years kept him out of the deepest valleys, but he felt flat, unfocused, disconnected from purpose. He slept poorly, relied on energy drinks to start his mornings, and by afternoon was either jittery or exhausted. He ate whatever was fast—fast food, snacks, pastries—and when stress rose, he ate more.

The Challenge: He didn't believe food mattered because he'd never seen it modeled. When you feel gray, it's hard to make bold changes.

The Intervention: We didn't make a bold change—we made a compassionate one. A two-week experiment:

- Two breakfast options (rotated):
    - Yogurt with berries, walnuts, olive oil drizzle
    - Eggs with spinach and whole grain toast

- Two lunch options:
  - Lentil soup with olive oil and fruit
  - Chickpea salad with tomatoes, cucumbers, herbs, lemon
- **Dinner template:** Protein, generous salad, grain, olive oil

We replaced energy drinks with water and green tea (caffeine without the crash). One 10-minute walk daily in the sun.

The Results

- **Week 1:** Sleep improved (stable glucose stops 2 AM brain alarms)
- **Week 3:** He felt hungry at breakfast—not nauseated or jittery, just clean hunger
- **Week 6:** Read a book for pleasure (first time in years)
- **Month 3:** Psychiatrist lowered medication dose; he was steadier, more motivated
- **Month 6:** "Food didn't cure me—it cleared enough fog that I could be reached"

The Science: David's recovery reflects the SMILES Trial: Mediterranean diet improved depression remission by 32%. Mechanisms: omega-3 fats help neurons communicate; steady glucose stabilizes mood, fermented foods and fiber reshape the microbiome and calm systemic inflammation that drives despair.

The Lesson: The science is not cold—it is a door opening in a room that felt dark.

CASE STUDY: Luisa's Cholesterol Defense

Background: Luisa, forty-seven, had a cholesterol profile that frightened her: high LDL despite a good dose of statin. Her father died at fifty-two of a heart attack. Fear lived under her busy days. She ate well compared to peers—little fried food, not many sweets—but she hadn't oriented her plate around foods that actively change lipid metabolism.

The Challenge: Despite medication, her LDL remained dangerously high. She needed food to work with her statin, not against it.

The Intervention: We built a polyphenol-rich, fiber-dense routine:

- Every morning: Green tea steeped 5 minutes while preparing oatmeal topped with blueberries and chopped walnuts
- Every afternoon: Apple and handful of almonds
- Lunch rotation: Lentil vegetable soup or sardine and arugula salad with olive oil and lemon
- Dinner: Chicken, fish, or beans + vegetables + whole grains + olive oil
- Treats: Pomegranate seeds over yogurt, dark chocolate in the freezer

The Results

- **Month 2:** LDL decreased noticeably, triglycerides down, HDL up
- **Month 4:** LDL dropped by 25%, clinician kept medication unchanged
- **Month 6:** Luisa felt both safer and stronger

The Science: Polyphenols turn down inflammatory gene expression (Nutrients, 2018). Omega-3s make cell membranes more fluid. Fiber captures bile acids and escorts them away. The numbers reflect cellular changes you cannot see—but you can direct every single day.

The Lesson: "It feels like I'm finally doing the part that belongs to me," Luisa said. Food became her agency, not her enemy.

CASE STUDY: Roberto's Post-Stroke Recovery

Background: Roberto, sixty-three, had survived a mild stroke that left him with a limp and terror he tried to hide. He took medications faithfully but wasn't convinced he could do more than hope.

The Challenge: Fear of the next stroke paralyzed him as much as the first one had.

The Intervention: We talked about Ikaria and Sardinia—about beans simmered with onions and olive oil, sourdough bread dipped in tomato and herbs, vegetables roasted until sweet, the purpose that grows when people eat together.

His kitchen became therapy:

- **Sunday meal PREP:** Pot of minestrone with beans and barley, tray of roasted vegetables with rosemary, container of chickpea salad, bowl of washed greens
- **Daily routine:** Switched bread to whole grain sourdough, walked after lunch around the block
- **Weekly ritual:** Invited his granddaughter to cook—made lentil patties and salmon, laughed when they failed at flipping the first one

The Results

- **Month 4:** Lab work pleased his neurologist—blood pressure controlled, lipids improved, weight down
- **Year 2:** No further events, brisker walk, more confidence Lasting impact: Family memory of the grandfather who made Sunday soup

The Science: the Ornish Lifestyle Trial proved that plant-based diets can reverse arterial narrowing. Roberto's kitchen was a clinic, and he was an active patient rather than a frightened passenger.

The Lesson: When I say food is medicine, I don't mean only molecules and pathways. I mean the rituals that lower stress hormones, the laughter that warms a table, the certainty that you are not helpless.

SECTION 3: PSYCHIATRY ON THE PLATE

In psychiatry, we discuss neurotransmitters and synapses—but the raw materials for those chemical conversations arrive on a fork and in a glass.

How Food Shapes Mental Health:

- Serotonin pathways depend on tryptophan availability and steady insulin response
- Dopamine signaling responds to omega-3 content in neuronal membranes
- GABA (calming neurotransmitter) is influenced by gut microbial metabolites that depend on fiber
- Magnesium calms the stress response
- Polyphenols protect neurons from oxidative stress
- Iron deficiency can masquerade as attention disorder

The Evidence:

Depression responds to anti-inflammatory, omega-3-rich diets. When people move from ultra-processed patterns to Mediterranean patterns, symptoms lessen; remission becomes more likely; relapse risk declines.

Anxiety lightens when blood sugar swings are minimized, caffeine moderated, and magnesium appears in greens, legumes, nuts, and seeds.

ADHD symptoms improve when breakfast contains protein; the day includes omega-3 sources and iron sufficiency, and hydration isn't an afterthought.

Bipolar disorder is complex, but depressive phases may soften with omega-3 supplementation and patterns that support sleep and stabilize circadian rhythms.

Trauma survivors benefit from anti-inflammatory diets that support gut integrity and reduce chemical signals that keep the nervous system on high alert.

Medication remains vital, and therapy is irreplaceable—but food is the terrain on which recovery stands. When patients tell me they want to feel like themselves again, food is one of the first places we find traction because it's a daily choice they control.

SECTION 4: THE PRACTICAL TOOLKIT

Building a Kitchen That Treats You Well

Stock this (so the healthy choice is the easy choice):

- Legumes Lentils, chickpeas, black beans, white beans (canned or dry for flexibility)
- Whole Grains Quinoa, oats, barley, brown rice, whole grain sourdough bread.
- Vegetables Leafy greens (spinach, kale, arugula), crucifers (broccoli, cauliflower, Brussels sprouts), peppers, carrots, onions, tomatoes
- Fruits Berries (fresh or frozen), citrus, apples, pomegranate, bananas
- Healthy Fats Extra virgin olive oil, walnuts, almonds, chia seeds, pumpkin seeds, ground flaxseed
- Protein Salmon, sardines (canned is fine), eggs, plain yogurt or kefir, tofu or tempeh
- Flavor Builders Garlic, onions, fresh herbs (rosemary, oregano, basil, parsley), spices (turmeric, cumin, cinnamon), lemon

Clear out (or move to the back):

- Sugar-sweetened beverages
- Refined white breads and crackers
- Processed meats
- Pastries and candies that trigger craving cycles

Batch Prep That Saves Your Week

Sunday routine (90 minutes):

1. Cook a pot of beans or lentils
2. Roast two trays of mixed vegetables with olive oil and herbs
3. Cook a grain (quinoa, barley, brown rice)
4. Boil a half-dozen eggs
5. Wash and spin a big bowl of greens
6. Mix a jar of lemon-olive oil dressing (3:1 ratio, salt, pepper)
7. Put fruit in a visible bowl
8. Move nuts and seeds to the front of a shelf
9. Keep a liter bottle of water within reach wherever you work

Result: Healthy meals are assembled in 10 minutes every week.

Quick Swaps That Deliver Without Deprivation

Instead...	Try this...
Soda	Lemon or lime water, sparkling water
Chips	Roasted chickpeas, nuts, air-popped popcorn
White bread	Whole grain sourdough
Creamy sauces	Olive oil + lemon + herbs
Fast food burger	10-minute skillet: onions + tomatoes + chickpeas + spinach + olive oil + bread
Ice cream	Frozen banana blended with berries

SECTION 5: THE 7-DAY STARTER PLAN

This plan teaches as it nourishes. Each day includes what to eat and why to eat it.

DAY 1: STABILIZE

MORNING Greek Yogurt Bowl: Plain yogurt + blueberries + walnuts + drizzle of honey (taper if transitioning from high sugar) Why: Protein steadies your morning; probiotics support gut-brain signaling; blueberries deliver anthocyanins that protect neurons and skin; walnuts provide omega-3 fatty acids that help your brain handle stress.

MIDDAY Turmeric Lentil Soup: Lentils + carrots + onions + garlic + tomatoes + olive oil + spinach at the end Why: This bowl feeds your microbiome, gives iron and folate, stabilizes glucose so your afternoon doesn't collapse. Eat a piece of fruit after (apple or orange).

EVENING Salmon with Quinoa & Broccoli: Pan-seared salmon + roasted broccoli with olive oil and lemon + quinoa Why: Salmon supplies DHA (omega-3 that supports mood and attention), quinoa is complete protein, roasted broccoli delivers sulforaphane, olive oil improves absorption of fat-soluble antioxidants.

DAILY PRACTICE Walk 10 minutes after lunch or dinner. Drink water in the afternoon.

DAY 2: MOMENTUM

MORNING Oatmeal Power Bowl: Oats + chia seeds + banana slices + cinnamon Why: Oats and chia lower cholesterol, banana brings potassium for blood pressure and mood; cinnamon adds flavor without sugar.

MIDDAY Mediterranean Chickpea Salad: Chickpeas + cucumbers + tomatoes + parsley + olive oil + lemon + a few olives Why: You can assemble this in 5 minutes if you keep canned chickpeas and chopped vegetables ready. Resistant starch in chickpeas feeds gut bacteria, supports steady energy.

EVENING Cod with Kale & Sweet Potato: Baked cod + kale sautéed in olive oil and garlic + roasted sweet potato Why: Cod is lean protein, kale brings vitamin K and magnesium, sweet potato supplies carotenoids for skin and immune health. If you crave dessert, have berries.

DAILY PRACTICE Replace afternoon coffee with green tea (if caffeine-sensitive). Notice your energy levels without crashes.

DAY 3: ATTENTION

MORNING Eggs with Greens: Scrambled eggs + spinach + whole grain sourdough toast Why: Protein in the morning improves attention (crucial for ADHD management). Spinach brings folate and magnesium that support neurotransmitter production.

MIDDAY Black Bean Bowl: Black beans + avocado + pico de gallo + lime + brown rice Why: Nicoya (a Blue Zones) thrives on beans and corn. This bowl gives steady energy and satisfaction without the crash.

EVENING Mediterranean Vegetable Bake: Eggplant + zucchini + peppers + tomatoes + onions tossed with olive oil and oregano, roasted until sweet, served with barley or brown rice Why: This is plant abundance, and it tastes like comfort.

DAILY PRACTICE Eat without screens at one meal. Notice flavors, textures, and how your body feels.

DAY 4: GUT-BRAIN CONNECTION

MORNING Probiotic Smoothie: Spinach + banana + pumpkin seeds + kefir + cooled green tea blended Why: L-theanine in green tea smooths caffeine's edges, pumpkin seeds bring magnesium, kefir brings diverse probiotics that influence mood via the gut-brain axis.

MIDDAY Sardinian Minestrone: Beans + barley + carrots + celery + cabbage or kale + rosemary + olive oil Why: This is longevity in a pot—a Sardinian staple. Have a side salad of arugula with olive oil and lemon.

EVENING Sardines on Toast: Whole grain toast + sardines + sliced tomato + roasted carrots on the side Why: Sardines are affordable omega-3s and calcium, tomatoes add lycopene, carrots add carotenoids.

DAILY PRACTICE Journal one sentence about how you felt after each meal. Patients often realize meals change mood within hours, not years.

DAY 5: ANTI-INFLAMMATORY

MORNING Flax Oatmeal: Oatmeal + ground flaxseed + apple slices + cinnamon Why: Flaxseed is a plant omega-3 source and provides lignans that may reduce breast cancer risk. Apples bring quercetin, an anti-inflammatory flavonoid.

MIDDAY Hummus Plate: Hummus + raw vegetables (carrots, peppers, cucumbers) + olives + whole grain pita Why: Chickpeas stabilize blood sugar, tahini offers calcium, olives provide anti-inflammatory polyphenols.

EVENING Roasted Chicken with Lentils: Roast chicken (or chickpea curry if plant-based) + arugula salad + lentils on the side Why: Arugula and leafy greens are high in nitrates that improve vascular flexibility. Lentils add folate, iron, slow-digesting carbs.

DAILY PRACTICE Replace dessert pastries with fresh fruit and a small square of dark chocolate (70%+ cacao). Dark chocolate polyphenols improve endothelial function.

DAY 6: STRENGTH & RECOVERY

MORNING Kefir Berry Bowl: Kefir + blueberries + chia seeds Why: Probiotics repair gut health after stress, blueberries protect neurons, chia stabilizes glucose for sustained energy.

MIDDAY Chickpea Turmeric Stew: Chickpeas + spinach + turmeric + cumin + tomatoes Why: Chickpeas provide satiety, spinach provides iron, turmeric reduces inflammation through curcumin.

EVENING Salmon with Peppers & Quinoa: Grilled salmon + roasted bell peppers and onions + quinoa Why: Perfect balance of protein, omega-3s, fiber, and antioxidants. Athletes in studies recover faster with anti-inflammatory foods like these.

DAILY PRACTICE Add 20 minutes of resistance training today (body-weight or weight). Food provides the building blocks; strength keeps aging at bay.

DAY 7: REFLECTION & RENEWAL

MORNING Chia Pudding: Chia seeds + almond milk + pomegranate seeds + chopped walnuts (prepared night before) Why: Pomegranate seeds are rich in punicalagins (antioxidants that reduce vascular inflammation), walnuts supply omega-3s, chia stabilizes glucose.

MIDDAY Probiotic Veggie Wrap: Whole grain wrap + avocado + black beans + sautéed peppers and onions + spoonful of sauerkraut + lime Why: Perfect gut-brain meal—probiotics, fiber, plant protein, potassium.

EVENING Mediterranean Grain Bowl: Quinoa + chickpeas + cucumbers + tomatoes + herbs + olive oil + lemon + optional feta or dairy-free crumble Why: This is the ultimate prevention bowl—the exact combination of foods associated with reduced cardiovascular and cancer risk. Eat slowly. Notice that you are not deprived. This is pleasure without the crash.

DAILY PRACTICE Write two sentences about what changed this week. Better sleep? More energy? Fewer cravings? Even the smallest win is proof that your body is responsive and alive.

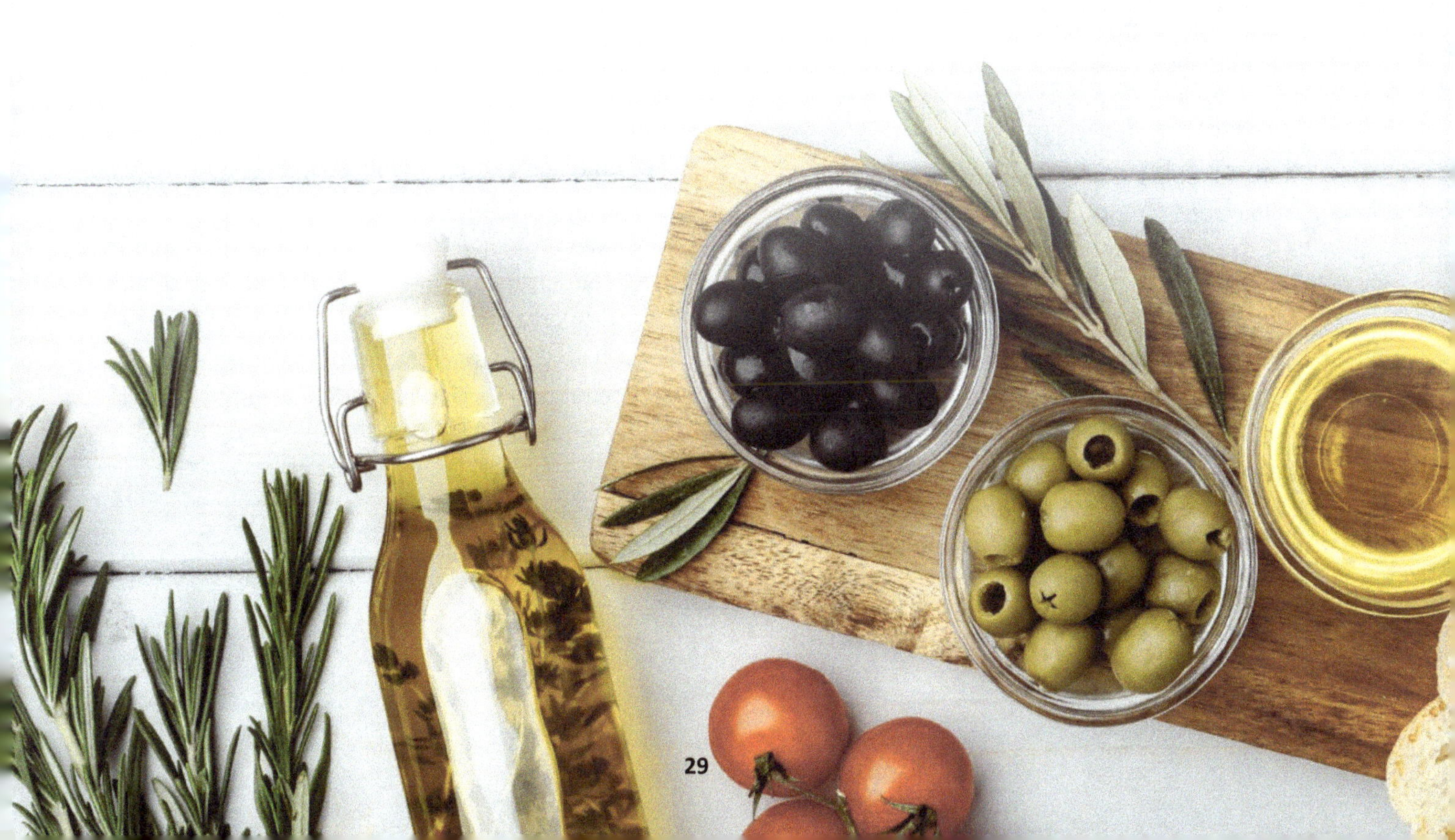

TURMERIC LENTIL SOUP (Featured Recipe)

A pot that anchors the week with anti-inflammatory power.

SERVES: 6 | **PREP:** 15 min | **COOK:** 40 min

WHY IT WORKS *This Sardinian-inspired soup delivers soluble fiber that lowers cholesterol, protein that stabilizes blood sugar, and turmeric curcumin that calms systemic inflammation. Perfect for meal prep—it supports heart health, mental clarity, and gut healing.*

INGREDIENTS

For the base:

- 1 cup brown or green lentils, rinsed
- 1 onion, chopped
- 2 carrots, diced
- 2 celery stalks, diced
- 3 garlic cloves, minced
- 1 can (14 oz) crushed tomatoes
- 6 cups vegetable broth or water

For seasoning:

- 3 tablespoons extra virgin olive oil
- 1 teaspoon turmeric powder
- ½ teaspoon black pepper (activates curcumin)
- 1 teaspoon ground cumin
- Salt to taste

To finish:

- 2 cups spinach or kale, chopped
- Juice of 1 lemon
- Extra olive oil for drizzling

METHOD

1. Heat olive oil in a large pot over medium heat. Sauté onion, carrot, and celery until softened (5-7 minutes).
2. Add garlic, turmeric, black pepper, and cumin. Stir until fragrant (1 minute).
3. Add tomatoes, lentils, and broth. Bring to a boil, then reduce to simmer.
4. Cook uncovered for 30-40 minutes until lentils are tender.
5. Stir in greens during the last 2 minutes until wilted.
6. Remove from heat, add lemon juice, and drizzle with olive oil before serving.

THE SCIENCE The Lancet (2019): Lentils' soluble fiber lowers LDL cholesterol by 5-10%. Turmeric's curcumin reduces inflammatory markers like CRP (American Journal of Clinical Nutrition, 2016). Black pepper increases curcumin absorption by 2,000%.

NUTRITIONAL HIGHLIGHTS ~250 calories per serving | Rich in: Fiber (12g), Folate, Iron, Magnesium

VARIATIONS

- Creamier texture: Blend 1 cup of soup and stir back in
- Extra protein: Add quinoa in the last 15 minutes
- Mediterranean twist: Top with crumbled feta and fresh oregano
- STORAGE Refrigerate up to 5 days. It freezes beautifully for 3 months. Reheat gently, adding water if needed to thin.

POMEGRANATE SALMON (Featured Recipe)

Polyphenols meet omega-3s in a celebration of flavor and healing.

SERVES: 4 | **PREP:** 10 min | **COOK:** 15 min

WHY IT WORKS *This dish unites anti-inflammatory fats with powerful antioxidants. Cancer survivors and heart patients benefit from this combination—it feels like celebration food but functions as therapy.*

INGREDIENTS

For the salmon:

- 4 salmon fillets (4-6 oz each)
- 2 tablespoons extra virgin olive oil
- Salt and pepper to taste
- 1 lemon, sliced

For serving:

- 3 cups fresh spinach
- 1 cup pomegranate seeds (arils)
- ¼ cup fresh parsley, chopped
- 2 tablespoons olive oil
- Juice of ½ lemon

METHOD

1. Preheat oven to 375°F (190°C).
2. Rub salmon fillets with 1 tablespoon of olive oil, salt, and pepper.
3. Place lemon slices on top.
4. Bake for 12-15 minutes until salmon is cooked through (flakes easily with a fork).
5. While salmon bakes, heat remaining olive oil in a large skillet over medium heat. Add spinach and sauté until just wilted (2 minutes). Add lemon juice.
6. Plate spinach, top with salmon, scatter pomegranate seeds, and finish with fresh parsley.

THE SCIENCE Salmon provides DHA, an omega-3 that reduces arrhythmia and stabilizes mood (JAMA, 2012). Pomegranate seeds are rich in punicalagins, shown to reduce arterial plaque (Atherosclerosis, 2015). Spinach supplies iron and folate for red blood cell health.

NUTRITIONAL HIGHLIGHTS ~380 calories per serving | Rich in: Omega-3s (2,000mg), Vitamin K, Iron, Polyphenols

VARIATIONS

- Budget-friendly: Use sardines on whole grain toast topped with pomegranate seeds
- Spice it up: Add a pinch of cumin and coriander to the spinach
- Make ahead: Cook salmon, refrigerate, and serve cold over salad

STORAGE Refrigerate cooked salmon for up to 3 days. Best fresh, but leftovers work beautifully in salads.

CLOSING: YOUR FIRST PRESCRIPTION LIVES IN YOUR KITCHEN

When I gave up sugar at fourteen, I thought I was giving up. It turned out I was claiming something—energy that didn't crash, skin that aged more slowly, mornings that felt steady, a mind that could focus, a body that could carry me through clinics and call nights and hard choices.

Decades later, I can say with conviction: food is not a side project. It is a central line into your future.

If your family history reads like mine did—strokes, heart attacks, pills handed down like heirlooms—you are not condemned. You can rewrite the story by:

- Stocking a pantry that serves you
- Cooking simple food that tastes like home
- Drinking water when your body asks for it
- Building a week that includes beans, greens, olive oil, and a walk in the sun

If your mood has been gray for so long that you've forgotten colors, know that food will not replace therapy or medication—but it will give both a foundation. It will lower the volume on inflammation, stabilize the swings, make mornings more navigable, and return a sense of control.

Food changes numbers on a lab report, and it also changes the way you feel in your life:

- It lets a grandmother climb stairs without stopping
- It lets a student sit through an exam with a present mind
- It lets a parent end the day without the 3 PM headache
- It lets an older man play on the floor with his granddaughter after a bowl of soup he made with his own hands

The prescription is not exotic—it's ordinary food: lentils and tomatoes, onions and greens, olive oil and lemon, whole grains and nuts, fish in modest portions, fruit that tastes like the place it grew.

The plan is not punishment—it's an abundance.

You don't need to become a different person. You need to become the person who stocks a different kitchen and repeats a few simple decisions until they become who you are.

If I could choose collard greens over cake at fourteen because I wanted a different ending than my family's, you can choose:

- A breakfast that steadies you
- A lunch that carries you
- A dinner that repairs you
- Water in a glass when the afternoon turns harsh

Start with one day, then one week, then one month. The body notices. The brain notices. The numbers notice. The people who love you will notice.

You will notice most of all.

This is the first prescription, written not in ink but in the meals you make and share.

Take it daily, and watch your life lengthen, soften, and brighten.

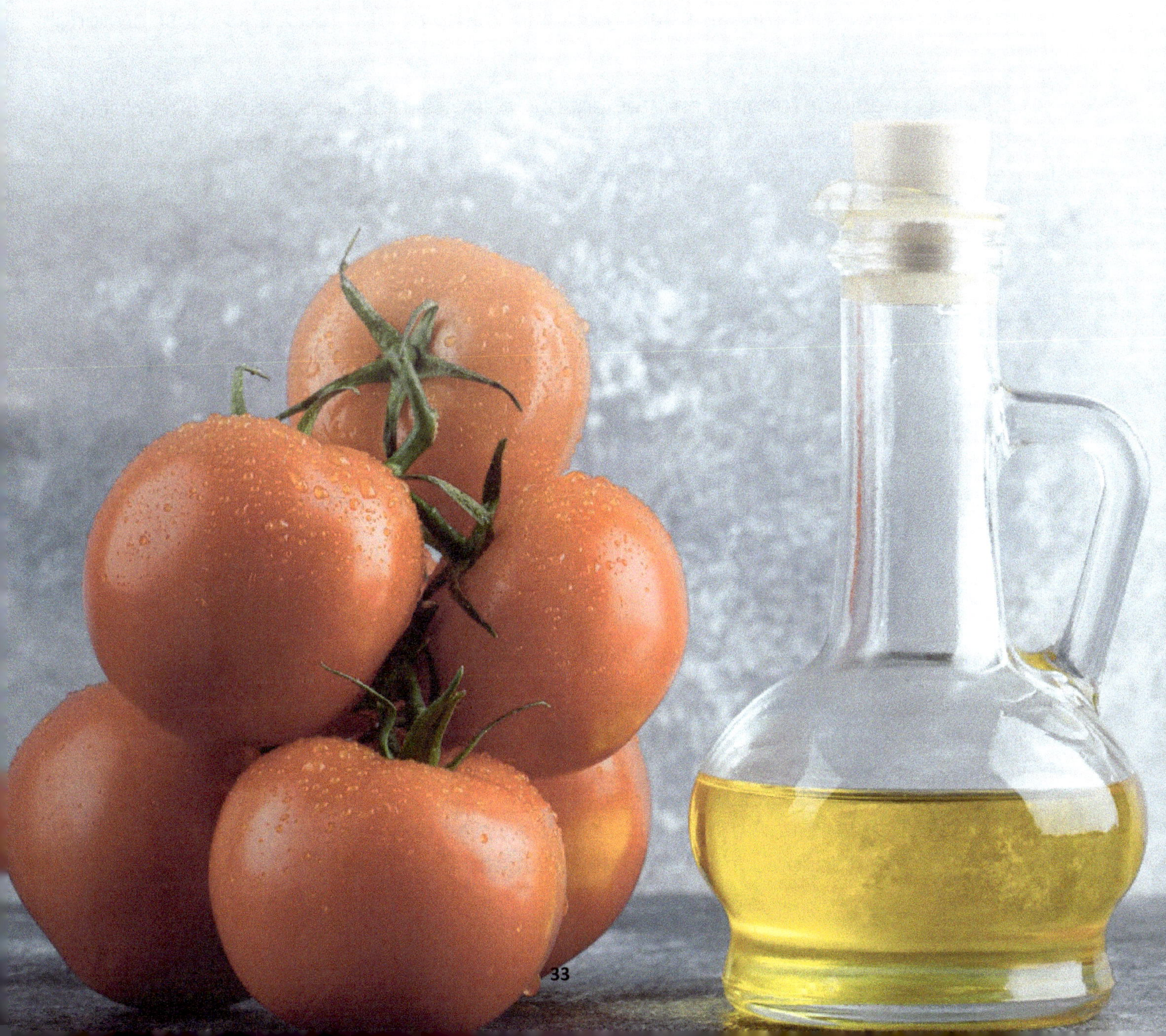

CHAPTER 2

Prevention Before Prescription

Food as the Shield

Prevention is quiet. It rarely makes headlines. It doesn't create drama in an emergency room. Yet prevention is the strongest medicine we have, and food is its most powerful form.

For decades, medicine focused on intervention—pills after diagnosis, surgery after disease, therapy after breakdown. But the most profound medical achievement isn't fixing what's broken. It's preventing the break in the first place.

Consider the numbers:

- 30% reduction in heart attacks with Mediterranean eating (PREDIMED, 2013)
- 58% reduction in diabetes with lifestyle change (Diabetes Prevention Program, 2002)
- 50% of cancers preventable through food and lifestyle (World Cancer Research Fund, 2018)
- 53% reduction in Alzheimer's risk with MIND diet adherence (Rush University, 2015)

These aren't small numbers. They represent parents who see their children graduate, survivors who live decades longer, older adults who preserve memory and independence.

But here's the challenge: prevention is invisible. Nobody wakes up saying, "Today I did not have a heart attack." Prevention works silently—in arteries that stay open, neurons that remain sharp, skin that holds its elasticity. It works in the absence of disease.

That invisibility is why so many dismiss prevention. Pills feel tangible; surgeries feel dramatic. But what is more powerful: opening a clogged artery, or never letting it clog in the first place?

Food is not a supplement to medicine. It is the stage on which medicine is performed. Without food, medication cannot reach its full effect.

SECTION 1: CARDIOVASCULAR DISEASE & DIET

Cardiovascular disease remains the single largest killer worldwide, responsible for 18 million deaths annually (WHO, 2022). Despite incredible progress in stents, bypass surgeries, and medications like statins, the fact remains: most of this disease is preventable.

What the Evidence Shows

The PREDIMED Trial (2013)

This landmark study, published in the New England Journal of Medicine, enrolled over 7,400 adults at high cardiovascular risk. Participants were randomly assigned to:

1. Mediterranean diet + extra virgin olive oil
2. Mediterranean diet + mixed nuts
3. Low-fat control diet

After just under five years, researchers stopped the study early because the Mediterranean groups had approximately 30% lower risk of heart attack, stroke, or cardiovascular death compared to the low-fat plan.

This wasn't a small observational suggestion. This was a randomized, controlled trial—the kind of gold-standard evidence normally reserved for drug approval. And yet, instead of a pill, the intervention was olive oil, nuts, beans, fish, and vegetables.

The Fiber Connection

A meta-analysis in The Lancet (2019), combining data from 185 studies, found that people consuming the highest levels of dietary fiber had a 15-30% reduction in both cardiovascular and all-cause mortality compared to those eating the least fiber.

To put that in perspective: switching white bread for whole grain bread, or trading soda for beans and fruit, can shift the arc of life and death.

Why Food Matters for the Heart

The mechanisms are powerful and multiple:

- Plant-based diets lower LDL cholesterol (the "bad" cholesterol that clogs arteries)
- Antioxidants in fruits and vegetables reduce oxidative stress on the vascular lining
- Omega-3 fatty acids reduce arrhythmias and stabilize plaques
- Fiber lowers cholesterol, regulates blood sugar, reduces weight, and lowers blood pressure simultaneously

The Olive Oil Evidence

The Journal of the American College of Cardiology (2020) analyzed over 90,000 U.S. adults and found that people who used olive oil regularly—just half a tablespoon daily—had:

- 14% lower risk of cardiovascular disease
- 21% lower risk of coronary heart disease

Replacing butter and margarine with olive oil shifted outcomes in measurable ways.

These numbers mean fewer funerals. They mean more grandparents watching their grandchildren graduate. They mean more lives extended not by machines in an ICU, but by lentil soup, sautéed greens, and bowls of beans.

CASE STUDY: Eduardo's Diabetes Prevention

Background: Eduardo, forty-four, was a quiet accountant who sat for long hours at his desk. He wasn't overweight by appearance, but his lab work told another story: fasting glucose of 112 mg/dL (prediabetes range). His father had lost his leg to diabetic complications. His uncle had been on dialysis before dying at sixty. Eduardo carried those images like a shadow.

The Challenge: His daily routine revealed the problem:

- Breakfast: White bread with butter and sweetened coffee
- Lunch: Fast food—fried chicken sandwiches, sodas, chips
- Dinner: Red meat, white rice, very few vegetables
- Daily: Three cans of soda
- Never: A bean salad

He had two paths: continue until glucose hit diabetic levels and start medication or intervene now with food.

The Intervention: We started with one change: soda. Eduardo replaced every sweetened drink with water (sometimes flavored with lemon or lime). He resisted at first, complaining of fatigue and cravings, but within two weeks felt less bloated.

The Results

- **Month 2:** We restructured breakfast—oats cooked with cinnamon, handful of walnuts, blueberries. He laughed at first, saying it felt "too American," but soon looked forward to it.
- **Month 3:** Lunch shifted from fried sandwiches to bean salads with olive oil, tomato, cucumber, and parsley. Dinner became a plate half-filled with vegetables, palm-sized protein, whole grains. Lost 7 pounds, energy steadier

- **Month 6:** Fasting glucose 94 mg/dL (normal), blood pressure dropped slightly, triglycerides improved, wife said he seemed less irritable

Quote: "I never believed food could change my numbers. I thought it was only medicine."

The Science: Eduardo's transformation mirrors the Diabetes Prevention Program (DPP, 2002): lifestyle changes cut diabetes risk by 58%, twice the effect of metformin.

The Lesson: By following the evidence—fiber for glucose control, omega-3s for inflammation, olive oil for vascular health—he reversed a trajectory that looked inevitable. His father's story no longer had to be his own.

CASE STUDY: Samuel's Heart Disease Reversal

Background: Samuel, sixty-one, had already survived one angina attack. His cholesterol was high, pressure uncontrolled, and weight creeping upward. "I feel like my heart is a ticking bomb," he admitted.

The Challenge: Despite medications, his cardiovascular risk remained dangerously high. He needed food to work with his medications, not against them.

The Intervention: We started simple:

- Olive oil instead of butter (everywhere)
- Oats for breakfast (with walnuts and berries)
- Beans at least 4x weekly (in soups, salads, as side dishes)
- Roasted vegetables and nuts instead of processed snacks
- Fish 2x weekly (salmon or sardines)

The Results

- **Month 3:** LDL cholesterol dropped 25 points
- **Month 6:** Could walk a mile without chest pain Year 1: Cardiologist reduced medications

Quote: "I thought heart disease was my family destiny. Now I know it's not written in stone."

The Science: Samuel's transformation echoed PREDIMED findings: diet changes heart outcomes as powerfully as interventions. The Lyon Diet Heart Study showed a 50-70% reduction in recurrent cardiac events with Mediterranean-style eating.

The Lesson: Heart disease did not disappear overnight, but Samuel proved what countless studies affirm: coronary artery disease can be slowed, stabilized, and in some cases partially reversed through comprehensive lifestyle change. The stent opened his artery, but the food kept it open.

SECTION 2: DIABETES & FOOD

The diabetes epidemic is one of the most pressing global health issues. More than 422 million people worldwide live with diabetes, and type 2 diabetes accounts for the vast majority. But type 2 diabetes is not inevitable. It is overwhelmingly a lifestyle—and therefore, preventable.

The Landmark Evidence

The Diabetes Prevention Program (DPP)

Published in the New England Journal of Medicine (2002), this study followed more than 3,200 adults with prediabetes. Participants were assigned to:

1. Intensive lifestyle change (diet + exercise)
2. Metformin medication
3. Placebo

The results stunned the medical world: after three years, the lifestyle group had a 58% lower incidence of diabetes, compared with a 31% reduction for metformin.

In other words, food and exercise worked twice as well as the leading medication.

Plant-Based Protection

A 2019 study in PLOS Medicine analyzed dietary patterns and found that adherence to a plant-based diet rich in whole grains, fruits, vegetables, nuts, and legumes was associated with a 23% lower risk of type 2 diabetes.

Conversely, each additional daily serving of processed red meat increased risk by 30-40% (Harvard School of Public Health, 2018).

Why Food Prevents Diabetes

The mechanisms are clear:

1. Diets high in refined starches and sugars spike blood sugar, damage insulin signaling, and drive fat deposition in the liver
2. Over time, this creates insulin resistance—the engine of type 2 diabetes
3. Diets rich in fiber slow glucose absorption
4. Antioxidants and omega-3s reduce the inflammatory state that underlies insulin resistance

In human terms: A breakfast of soda and white bread pushes the pancreas to exhaustion. A breakfast of oatmeal, walnuts, and berries gives the pancreas room to breathe.

Multiply that choice over 365 days, and you are either protecting yourself from diabetes or walking directly toward it.

CASE STUDY: Lisa's Diabetes Reversal

Background: Lisa, fifty-two, worked as a nurse. Her diet was quick cafeteria food, often processed. She developed type 2 diabetes and had been taking insulin for five years. She thought diabetes was a lifelong sentence.

The Challenge: Despite insulin, her HbA1c was 9.1% (poorly controlled). She felt defeated, exhausted, and trapped.

The Intervention: Under medical supervision, she joined a structured lifestyle program emphasizing plant-based eating and walking:

- High-fiber meals: Beans, lentils, whole grains at every meal
- Vegetables: At least 5-7 servings daily
- Healthy fats: Olive oil, nuts, avocado
- Eliminated: Processed foods, sugary drinks, refined carbs
- Added: 30-minute daily walks

The Results

- **Month 6:** HbA1c dropped to 7.2%, insulin dose reduced.
- **Month 12:** HbA1c 5.8% (normal), completely off insulin, lost 30 pounds

Quote: "I never imagined I could be free of insulin. Food gave me my life back."

The Science: Lisa's case echoes Lancet Diabetes & Endocrinology (2020) findings: structured diet programs can reverse diabetes in up to 46% of patients.

The Lesson: Type 2 diabetes is not always a one-way street. With commitment and medical support, reversal is possible—and food is the primary tool.

SECTION 3: CANCER PREVENTION

Cancer is often described as a genetic disease, and it's true that mutations drive tumor growth. But lifestyle factors strongly influence both cancer risk and outcomes.

The World Cancer Research Fund (2018) estimates that 30-50% of cancers could be prevented through diet, activity, and lifestyle.

The Fiber-Cancer Connection

High-fiber diets are consistently associated with lower rates of colorectal cancer. A study in the Journal of the National Cancer Institute (2015) found that people with the highest fiber intake had a 20-30% reduced risk of colorectal cancer compared to those with the lowest.

Fiber doesn't just pass through the gut—it ferments into short-chain fatty acids like butyrate, which have anti-inflammatory and even anti-tumor properties.

Cruciferous Vegetables

Broccoli, cauliflower, kale, and Brussels sprouts are rich in glucosinolates.

These break down into bioactive chemicals like sulforaphane, which can:

- Detoxify carcinogens
- Promote apoptosis (programmed cell death that stops cancer cells from spreading)

In laboratory studies, sulforaphane has been shown to suppress tumor growth in breast and prostate cancer models.

The Processed Meat Warning

Excessive processed meat consumption is classified as a Group 1 carcinogen by the World Health Organization—in the same category as smoking and asbestos (not because the risk is identical, but because the evidence is that strong).

Every 50 grams of processed meat per day increases colorectal cancer risk by about 18%.

Sugar and Cancer

While not a direct carcinogen, sugar contributes to:

- Obesity
- Inflammation
- Insulin resistance

All factors that increase cancer risk.

Food is not a guarantee, but it is a lever. It means that someone like Helena, a breast cancer survivor, can choose a diet of beans, greens, flaxseed, and green tea—and statistically improve her odds of long-term survival.

CASE STUDY: Helena's Breast Cancer Defense

Background: Helena, fifty-two, recently completed chemotherapy and radiation for breast cancer. She was thin, pale, and afraid. Her oncologist had discussed tamoxifen and surveillance imaging, but Helena wanted something more: "How do I rebuild my body from the inside?"

The Challenge: Her diet reflected what many busy professionals fall into:

- Skipped breakfast
- Pastries with coffee mid-morning
- Sandwiches at lunch
- Late dinners of pasta with cream sauces
- Vegetables once or twice a week
- Alcohol: two glasses of wine most nights

The Intervention: We started with education: diet is not a cure for cancer, but evidence shows it reduces recurrence risk. She committed to three food strategies:

1. Daily cruciferous vegetables: Broccoli, kale, arugula, Brussels sprouts
2. Flaxseed: Two tablespoons daily (sprinkled on yogurt or oatmeal), providing lignans with weak estrogenic effects that help modulate hormonal signaling
3. Alcohol reduction: Wine limited to once a week

We also added:

- Blueberries (antioxidants)
- Beans (fiber, plant protein)
- Green tea (polyphenols)
- Salmon twice weekly (omega-3s)

The Results

- Month 3: She described vegetables as "no longer boring"—roasted broccoli with garlic and olive oil, kale blended into smoothies, lentil curries with turmeric
- Month 6: Regained lean weight, fatigue lessened, hot flashes reduced
- **Year 1:** Cancer-free, feeling "stronger than before treatment"
- Year 5: Still cancer-free

Quote: "Food gave me back a sense of control. I couldn't stop the cancer from coming, but I can choose what I eat every day. That choice makes me feel like I'm building a wall between me and recurrence."

The Science: A 2017 review in Breast Cancer Research demonstrated that women with higher intakes of fiber, cruciferous vegetables, and phytoestrogens had lower recurrence rates and improved survival.

The Lesson: Helena's story proves that while food cannot cure cancer, it can shift the odds significantly—and give patients agency in their healing.

SECTION 4: SKIN, HAIR, AGING & NUTRITION

Prevention is visible on the outside as much as the inside.

Skin Aging

High sugar diets accelerate the process of glycation, in which sugar molecules attach to collagen and elastin, making skin stiffer and more prone to wrinkles.

Research in the Journal of Dermatological Science (2017) confirms that advanced glycation end products (AGEs) from diet contribute to visible skin aging.

Antioxidants, in contrast, protect skin from ultraviolet damage and oxidative stress:

- Beta-carotene from carrots and sweet potatoes
- Lycopene from tomatoes
- Vitamin C from citrus and berries

All contribute to skin elasticity and brightness.

Hair Health

Hair also responds to diet:

- Iron deficiency (common in women) contributes to hair thinning
- Omega-3s reduce scalp inflammation and support follicle growth

In one study published in Dermato-Endocrinology (2018), women who took a supplement containing omega-3s and antioxidants experienced significant improvements in hair density and diameter compared with placebo.

Nails

Brittle nails often signal deficiencies in protein, iron, or biotin. Diets rich in legumes, eggs, nuts, and seeds restore strength and growth.

Biological Aging

Most profoundly, diet slows biological aging itself.

A 2021 study in The American Journal of Clinical Nutrition found that plant-rich diets were associated with longer telomeres—the protective caps on chromosomes that shorten with age.

In other words, beans, greens, nuts, and olive oil slow the clock at the cellular level.

CASE STUDY: Adriana's Skin & Hair Transformation

Background: Adriana, forty, worked in fashion. Yet her skin looked older than her age. She had brittle nails, thinning hair, and constant fatigue. Her labs were normal, but her diet told the story: pastries, fast food, little protein, no vegetables.

The Challenge: She wanted to look and feel better but didn't connect her diet to her appearance.

The Intervention: We explained glycation (sugar binding to collagen, stiffening skin and causing wrinkles) and antioxidants (molecules in fruits and vegetables that protect skin from UV and oxidative damage).

Her new routine:

- Breakfast: Chia pudding with berries and walnuts
- Lunch: Salmon with arugula and tomatoes
- Snacks: Almonds, apples, carrots
- Dinner: Lentil stew with turmeric and spinach

The Results

- **Month 3:** Skin had a glow her coworkers noticed, hair was shinier, nails stronger
- **Month 6:** She admitted she had doubted the connection between food and appearance but now saw it daily in the mirror

Quote: "My industry spends thousands on creams. I spent fifty dollars at the market and my face changed."

The Science: A study in the Journal of Dermatological Science (2017) confirmed that diets high in sugar accelerate collagen breakdown, while antioxidants slow aging. Another trial in Dermato-Endocrinology (2018) found that omega-3 and antioxidant supplementation improved hair density and thickness.

The Lesson: Beauty is not only skin-deep—it's plate-deep.

CASE STUDY: Camila's Hypertension Prevention

Camila, sixty-one, was a retired teacher. Her blood pressure was "borderline" on 142/88. She dreaded medications—her sister had taken pills for years and developed side effects. "Is there any way food can help me avoid that path?" she asked.

The Challenge: Her blood pressure was creeping into hypertensive range, but she wanted to try lifestyle before medication.

The Intervention: Yes. Studies in Hypertension (2019) show Mediterranean-style diets lower blood pressure significantly, sometimes enough to replace medications.

We built her food prescription:

- Beans 3x weekly (fiber, magnesium, potassium)
- Bananas or oranges daily (potassium)
- Olive oil as main fat (polyphenols relax blood vessels)
- Roasted vegetables instead of salty snacks
- Water with lemon instead of soda

She began batching beans and vegetables on Sundays. She discovered she enjoyed lentil salads with olive oil.

The Results

- **Month 2:** Blood pressure dropped to 130/82
- **Month 6:** Averaged 122/78, lost 12 pounds, felt "lighter, calmer, as if my body had exhaled"

Quote: "I never imagined beans and bananas could do what pills do."

The Science: JAMA (2019): DASH diet reduced systolic blood pressure by 11 mmHg in 8 weeks. Foods rich in potassium and polyphenols relax blood vessels and reduce vascular inflammation.

The Lesson: Camila still sees her doctor, but she controls her life through her kitchen.

SECTION 5: THE 7-DAY PREVENTIVE MEAL PLAN

GOAL: Reduce risk of heart disease, diabetes, cancer, cognitive decline, and premature aging FOCUS: Fiber, antioxidants, anti-inflammatory fats, stable glucose

DAY 1: STABILIZE THE FOUNDATION

MORNING Overnight Oats with Chia & Berries: Oats + chia seeds + blueberries + walnuts Why: Soluble fiber lowers cholesterol, chia stabilizes glucose and brings plant omega-3s, blueberries supply anthocyanins (shown in American Journal of Clinical Nutrition, 2019 to improve memory and protect neurons), walnuts add alpha-linolenic acid for brain and heart.

MIDDAY Lentil Soup with Greens: Lentils + spinach + tomatoes + onions + garlic + olive oil Why: High in fiber and protein for stable blood sugar, spinach adds magnesium (calms nervous system), olive oil enhances absorption of fat-soluble nutrients and lowers inflammation.

EVENING Salmon with Quinoa & Broccoli: Pan-seared salmon + quinoa + roasted broccoli Why: Salmon provides DHA (omega-3 essential for brain function and anti-arrhythmic protection), quinoa offers complete plant protein, broccoli delivers sulforaphane (linked to reduced cancer risk).

DAILY PRACTICE Walk 10-15 minutes after lunch or dinner. Studies show post-meal walking reduces blood sugar spikes significantly (Diabetes Care, 2016).

DAY 2: ENERGY WITHOUT SPIKES

MORNING Greek Yogurt Probiotic Bowl: Yogurt (or dairy-free kefir) + raspberries + almonds + cinnamon Why: Probiotics improve gut microbiome health (directly influences mood and immune function), raspberries are rich in vitamin C and fiber, almonds provide vitamin E and healthy fats, cinnamon lowers post-meal glucose response.

MIDDAY Chickpea Salad: Chickpeas + cucumbers + tomatoes + parsley + lemon + olive oil Why: Chickpeas are a Blue Zones staple, offering resistant starch that feeds beneficial gut bacteria. Parsley and lemon add vitamin C and phytochemicals.

EVENING Baked Cod with Kale & Sweet Potato: Baked cod + sautéed kale + roasted sweet potato Why: Cod is lean protein, kale brings vitamin K and folate, sweet potatoes provide beta-carotene for skin and immune resilience.

DAILY PRACTICE Swap soda or juice for sparkling water with lemon. Even modest reductions in sugary drink intake lower diabetes risk.

DAY 3: ATTENTION & MOOD SUPPORT

MORNING Eggs with Spinach & Sourdough: Scrambled eggs + spinach + whole grain sourdough toast Why: Eggs supply choline (essential for acetylcholine production, which improves memory and focus), spinach adds folate (linked to lower depression risk), whole grain sourdough provides slow-digesting carbs for steady energy.

MIDDAY Black Bean Bowl: Black beans + avocado + pico de gallo + lime + brown rice Why: Black beans stabilize blood sugar and provide magnesium, avocado adds potassium (lowers blood pressure), lime adds vitamin C and flavor.

EVENING Mediterranean Vegetable Bake: Roasted eggplant + zucchini + peppers + tomatoes + onions with olive oil and herbs, served with barley Why: Barley lowers cholesterol, roasted vegetables provide a spectrum of antioxidants, olive oil enhances nutrient absorption. This is the pattern seen in Ikaria, a Greek Blue Zones.

DAILY PRACTICE Take 5 minutes to eat mindfully at one meal. Chewing slowly lowers cortisol and improves digestion.

DAY 4: GUT-BRAIN CONNECTION

MORNING Probiotic Power Smoothie: Kefir + banana + spinach + pumpkin seeds + cooled green tea, blended Why: Kefir is rich in probiotics, banana provides prebiotic fiber, pumpkin seeds supply zinc and magnesium, green tea offers L-theanine (smooths caffeine's stimulating effect).

MIDDAY Sardinian Minestrone: Beans + barley + carrots + kale + rosemary + olive oil Why: This soup is a longevity staple. Beans and barley provide plant protein and fiber, kale supports detoxification, olive oil brings antioxidants.

EVENING Sardines on Toast: Whole grain toast + sardines + tomatoes + roasted carrots Why: Sardines are one of the most nutrient-dense, affordable foods: omega-3s, vitamin D, calcium, and protein. Carrots supply beta-carotene for vision and skin.

DAILY PRACTICE Journal one sentence about how you feel after each meal. Patients often realize meals change mood within hours, not years.

DAY 5: LOWERING INFLAMMATION

MORNING Flax Oatmeal: Oatmeal + ground flaxseed + apple slices + cinnamon Why: Flaxseed adds lignans (may reduce breast cancer risk) and provides omega-3s. Apples bring quercetin, an anti-inflammatory flavonoid.

MIDDAY Hummus Plate: Hummus + raw vegetables (carrots, peppers, cucumbers) + olives + whole grain pita Why: Chickpeas stabilize blood sugar, tahini offers calcium, olives provide anti-inflammatory polyphenols.

EVENING Roasted Chicken with Lentils: Roast chicken (or chickpea curry) + arugula salad + lentils Why: Arugula and leafy greens are high in nitrates that improve vascular flexibility. Lentils add folate, iron, and slow-digesting carbs.

DAILY PRACTICE Replace dessert pastries with fresh fruit and a small square of dark chocolate (70%+ cacao). Dark chocolate polyphenols improve endothelial function.

DAY 6: STRENGTH & RECOVERY

MORNING Kefir Berry Bowl: Kefir + blueberries + chia seeds Why: Probiotics repair gut health after stress, blueberries protect neurons, chia stabilizes glucose for sustained energy.

MIDDAY Chickpea Turmeric Stew: Chickpeas + spinach + turmeric + cumin + tomatoes Why: Chickpeas provide satiety, spinach provides iron, turmeric reduces inflammation through curcumin.

EVENING Grilled Salmon with Quinoa & Peppers: Grilled salmon + roasted bell peppers and onions + quinoa Why: Perfect balance of protein, omega-3s, fiber, and antioxidants. Athletes in studies recover faster with anti-inflammatory foods like these.

DAILY PRACTICE Add 20 minutes of resistance training today. Food provides the building blocks; strength keeps aging at bay.

DAY 7: REFLECTION & RENEWAL

MORNING Chia Pudding: Chia seeds (prepared night before with almond milk) + pomegranate seeds + walnuts Why: Pomegranate seeds are rich in punicalagins (antioxidants that reduce vascular inflammation), walnuts supply omega-3s, chia stabilizes glucose.

MIDDAY Probiotic Veggie Wrap: Whole grain wrap + avocado + black beans + sautéed peppers and onions + sauerkraut + lime Why: Perfect gut-brain meal—probiotics, fiber, plant protein, and potassium.

EVENING Mediterranean Grain Bowl: Quinoa + chickpeas + cucumbers + tomatoes + herbs + olive oil + lemon + optional feta Why: This is the ultimate prevention bowl—the exact combination of foods associated with reduced cardiovascular and cancer risk.

DAILY PRACTICE Write down three changes you noticed this week: better sleep, more energy, fewer cravings. Even the smallest shifts prove your body is responding.

SECTION 6: SEVEN PREVENTION RECIPES

1. TURMERIC LENTIL SOUP
2. POMEGRANATE SALMON

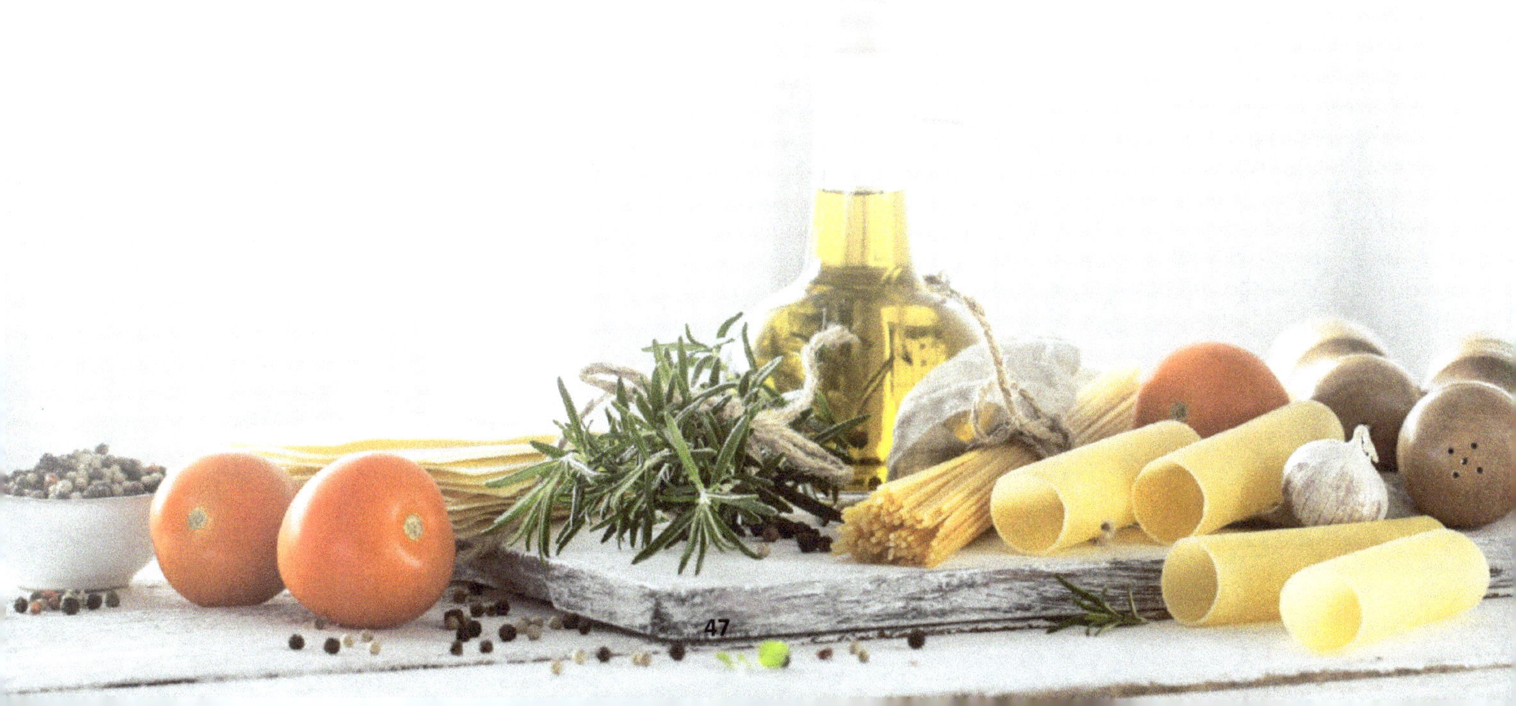

3. MEDITERRANEAN GRAIN BOWL (Featured Recipe)

The everyday hero that proves prevention can be assembled in 10 minutes.

SERVES: 4 | **PREP:** 10 min (if grains pre-cooked) | **COOK:** 0 min

WHY IT WORKS *Blue Zones families eat bowls like this several times weekly. The components are simple—beans, grains, vegetables, herbs, olive oil—but the combination delivers complete protein, resistant starch for gut health, polyphenols for cardiovascular protection, and steady energy without crashes.*

INGREDIENTS

For the base:

- 2 cups cooked quinoa or barley (cooled)
- 1 can (15 oz) chickpeas, drained and rinsed

For the vegetables:

- 1 cucumber, diced
- 1 cup cherry tomatoes, halved
- ½ red onion, thinly sliced
- ½ cup Kalamata olives, pitted

For the dressing:

- 3 tablespoons extra virgin olive oil
- Juice of 1 lemon
- Salt and pepper to taste
- Fresh parsley and mint, chopped

Optional:

- ¼ cup crumbled feta (or dairy-free alternative)

METHOD

1. In a large bowl, combine quinoa or barley with chickpeas.
2. Add cucumber, tomatoes, onion, and olives.
3. In a small bowl, whisk together olive oil, lemon juice, salt, and pepper.
4. Pour dressing over grain mixture and toss gently.
5. Fold in fresh herbs.
6. Top with feta if desired.
7. Serve at room temperature or chilled.

THE SCIENCE Chickpeas provide resistant starch that lowers glucose (Diabetes Care, 2018). Quinoa supplies all nine essential amino acids. Tomatoes bring lycopene (antioxidant that reduces prostate cancer risk in Cancer Epidemiology Biomarkers & Prevention, 2016). Olive oil polyphenols improve endothelial function.

NUTRITIONAL HIGHLIGHTS ~380 calories per serving | Rich in: Fiber (11g), Protein (12g), Polyphenols, B-vitamins

VARIATIONS

- Winter version: Swap fresh vegetables for roasted ones
- Extra satiety: Add sliced avocado
- More protein: Top with grilled chicken or tofu

STORAGE Refrigerate up to 4 days. Best if dressing is added just before serving, but can be dressed ahead for meal prep.

4. SARDINIAN MINESTRONE (Featured Recipe)

Longevity in a pot—the soup that feeds Sardinian centenarians.

SERVES: 8 | **PREP:** 15 min | **COOK:** 50 min

WHY IT WORKS *This soup appears repeatedly in the lives of Sardinian centenarians because it's inexpensive, nourishing, and deeply satisfying. It combines legumes and grains for broader amino acid profiles, fiber for cholesterol reduction, and rosemary for antioxidants that make simple food feel abundant.*

INGREDIENTS

For the base:

- 3 tablespoons extra virgin olive oil
- 1 onion, diced
- 2 carrots, diced
- 2 celery stalks, diced
- 3 garlic cloves, minced

For the soup:

- 1 can (15 oz) white beans or mixed beans
- ½ cup pearl barley
- 1 can (14 oz) diced tomatoes
- 6 cups vegetable broth or water
- 2 cups chopped cabbage or kale
- 1 teaspoon dried rosemary
- 1 teaspoon dried thyme
- Salt and pepper to taste

To finish:

- Extra olive oil for drizzling
- Fresh parsley, chopped
- Optional: spoonful of pesto per bowl

METHOD

1. Heat olive oil in a large pot over medium heat. Sauté onion, carrot, and celery until softened (6-8 minutes).
2. Add garlic and stir for 1 minute until fragrant.
3. Add beans, barley, tomatoes, and broth. Bring to a boil.
4. Reduce heat and simmer for 40 minutes, stirring occasionally.
5. Add cabbage or kale and herbs in the last 10 minutes.
6. Season with salt and pepper.

- Serve in bowls with a drizzle of olive oil and fresh parsley.
- Optional: Stir in a spoonful of pesto at the table for extra flavor.

THE SCIENCE Barley lowers cholesterol and improves gut microbiota (Nutrients, 2018). Beans supply folate and resistant starch. Cruciferous greens activate detoxification enzymes that reduce cancer risk. Rosemary adds aroma and antioxidants.

NUTRITIONAL HIGHLIGHTS ~220 calories per serving | Rich in: Fiber (9g), Protein (8g), Iron, Folate

VARIATIONS

- Extra vegetables: Add zucchini, green beans, or spinach
- Creamier: Mash some beans against the side of the pot
- Heartier: Add whole grain pasta in the last 10 minutes

STORAGE Refrigerates beautifully for 5 days. It freezes for 3 months. The flavors deepen overnight.

5. BLUEBERRY CHIA PUDDING (Featured Recipe)

Easy resilience—mornings won the night before.

SERVES: 4 | **PREP:** 5 min + overnight refrigeration

WHY IT WORKS *Mornings are won the night before, when breakfast is already waiting in the refrigerator. This simple pudding delivers omega-3s and fiber that stabilize glucose and mood, while berries' anthocyanins protect memory and slow cognitive decline.*

INGREDIENTS

- ½ cup chia seeds
- 2 cups almond milk (or milk of choice)
- 1 teaspoon vanilla extract
- Pinch of salt
- 1 cup fresh or frozen blueberries
- ¼ cup chopped walnuts
- Optional: 1-2 teaspoons honey or maple syrup

METHOD

1. In a large bowl or jar, whisk together chia seeds, milk, vanilla, and salt.
2. If using sweetener, add now and whisk to combine.
3. Divide mixture among 4 small jars or containers.
4. Refrigerate overnight (or at least 4 hours).
5. In the morning, top each serving with blueberries and walnuts.

THE SCIENCE Chia provides omega-3s and soluble fiber that stabilizes blood sugar. Blueberries improve memory and reduce oxidative stress (Nutrients, 2020). Walnuts add plant-based omega-3s (alpha-linolenic acid) and polyphenols that lower inflammation.

NUTRITIONAL HIGHLIGHTS ~240 calories per serving | Rich in: Fiber (11g), Omega-3s, Calcium, Antioxidants

VARIATIONS

- Chocolate version: Add 1 tablespoon cocoa powder
- Extra protein: Stir in 2 tablespoons Greek yogurt per serving
- Seasonal: Top with strawberries, raspberries, or sliced banana
- Warmth: Add cinnamon or cardamom

STORAGE Prepare up to 5 days in advance. Add toppings fresh each morning.

6. ANTI-INFLAMMATORY GOLDEN LENTILS (Featured Recipe)

Curcumin-powered comfort that calms the body from within.

SERVES: 6 | **PREP:** 10 min | **COOK:** 35 min

WHY IT WORKS *This dish combines the cholesterol-lowering power of lentils with turmeric anti-inflammatory curcumin. Perfect for anyone managing arthritis, heart disease, or chronic inflammation. It's comfort food that heals.*

INGREDIENTS

For the base:

- 2 tablespoons coconut oil or olive oil
- 1 onion, diced
- 3 garlic cloves, minced
- 1 tablespoon fresh ginger, grated

For the lentils:

- 1 cup red lentils, rinsed
- 1 can (14 oz) coconut milk
- 2 cups vegetable broth
- 2 teaspoons ground turmeric
- 1 teaspoon ground cumin
- ½ teaspoon black pepper (activates curcumin)
- 1 teaspoon salt

To finish:

- 2 cups fresh spinach
- Juice of 1 lime
- Fresh cilantro, chopped

METHOD

1. Heat oil in a large pot over medium heat. Sauté onion until softened (5 minutes).
2. Add garlic and ginger, stir for 1 minute until fragrant.
3. Add turmeric, cumin, and black pepper. Stir for 30 seconds.
4. Add lentils, coconut milk, and broth. Bring to a boil.
5. Reduce heat and simmer for 20-25 minutes until lentils are soft.
6. Stir in spinach until wilted.
7. Remove from heat, add lime juice.
8. Serve over brown rice or quinoa, garnished with fresh cilantro.

THE SCIENCE Turmeric's curcumin reduces inflammatory markers like CRP and IL-6 (Journal of Medicinal Food, 2016). Black pepper increases curcumin absorption by 2,000%. Lentils provide fiber and protein that stabilize blood sugar. Coconut milk adds medium-chain triglycerides (MCTs) that support brain health.

NUTRITIONAL HIGHLIGHTS ~280 calories per serving | Rich in: Fiber (8g), Protein (10g), Curcumin, Iron

VARIATIONS

- Extra vegetables: Add diced sweet potato or carrots
- Spicier: Add cayenne or red chili flakes
- Creamier: Use full-fat coconut milk

STORAGE Refrigerate up to 5 days. Freezes well for 3 months. Reheat gently, adding liquid if needed.

7. HEART-PROTECTING OLIVE OIL ROASTED VEGETABLES (Featured Recipe)

The sheet pan solution that wins the week.

SERVES: 6 | **PREP:** 15 min | **COOK:** 30 min

WHY IT WORKS *Most weeks are won because you cooked once and ate well three times. Roasting concentrates flavor, olive oil carries fat-soluble antioxidants, and these vegetables bring a spectrum of vitamins and phytochemicals that your skin, vessels, and brain recognize as support.*

INGREDIENTS

- Choose 8-10 cups total of:
- Carrots, cut into sticks
- Zucchini, chopped
- Bell peppers (red, yellow, orange), sliced
- Red onion, wedged
- Eggplant, cubed
- Broccoli florets
- Brussels sprouts, halved

For roasting:

- ¼ cup extra virgin olive oil
- 1 teaspoon salt
- ½ teaspoon black pepper
- 1 tablespoon fresh rosemary or thyme (or 1 teaspoon dried)

To finish:

- Juice of 1 lemon
- Extra drizzle of olive oil

METHOD

1. Preheat oven to 425°F (220°C).
2. Cut all vegetables into similar-sized pieces for roasting.
3. In a large bowl, toss vegetables with olive oil, salt, pepper, and herbs until well coated.
4. Spread in a single layer on two large baking sheets (don't overcrowd—they'll steam instead of roast).
5. Roast for 25-30 minutes, stirring halfway through, until edges are caramelized, and vegetables are tender.
6. Remove from oven, squeeze lemon juice over top, and drizzle with extra olive oil before serving.

THE SCIENCE Roasting at high heat preserves antioxidants while enhancing flavor through caramelization. Olive oil increases absorption of carotenoids (beta-carotene, lycopene) by up to 400% (American Journal of Clinical Nutrition, 2004). These vegetables provide fiber, vitamin C, folate, and polyphenols that protect cardiovascular health.

NUTRITIONAL HIGHLIGHTS ~150 calories per serving | Rich in: Fiber (6g), Vitamin C, Carotenoids, Polyphenols

VARIATIONS

- Complete meal: Toss with cooked chickpeas and serve with whole grain bread
- Mediterranean: Add olives and feta after roasting
- Spicy: Sprinkle with red pepper flakes before roasting
- Asian-inspired: Use sesame oil instead of olive oil, add ginger and garlic

STORAGE Refrigerate up to 5 days. Reheat in oven or eat cold in salads or wraps.

CLOSING: PREVENTION AS POWER

When people think of medicine, they imagine a white pill in a bottle or a procedure in a hospital. They imagine intervention after something has already gone wrong. Prevention is quieter. It rarely makes headlines. It doesn't create drama in an emergency room.

Yet prevention is the strongest medicine we have, and food is its most powerful form.

Science is no longer vague. It is consistent, global, and clear:

- Mediterranean dietary patterns lower cardiovascular risk by 30% (NEJM, 2013)
- Lifestyle change reduces diabetes incidence by 58%, far more than medication alone (Diabetes Prevention Program, 2002)
- Up to 50% of cancers are preventable through food and lifestyle (World Cancer Research Fund, 2018)
- Plant-rich diets triple depression remission compared with standard care (SMILES Trial, 2017)
- Following the MIND diet reduces Alzheimer's risk by 53% (Alzheimer's & Dementia, 2015)

These are not small numbers. They are life changing. They represent parents who see their children graduate, survivors who live decades longer, and older adults who preserve memory and independence.

But here is the challenge: prevention is invisible. Nobody wakes up saying, "Today I did not have a heart attack," or "Today I did not develop diabetes." Prevention works silently—in arteries that stay open, neurons that remain sharp, skin that holds elasticity. It works in the absence of disease.

In my own life, prevention began when I was fourteen. I saw the pattern in my family—strokes, heart attacks, hypertension, cholesterol medications lined up on nightstands. I read an article on sugar and aging, and I decided I wanted a different future.

I gave up sugar. I ate greens and beans when my friends laughed. I chose olive oil, lentils, collard greens, and whole grains. That choice carried me through medical school, through residency, through nights in hospitals when fatigue could have consumed me.

It was not luck. It was prevention.

And yet, prevention is not perfection. Eduardo, who reversed prediabetes, didn't eat perfectly every day. Helena, the cancer survivor, still had moments of indulgence. Camila, who lowered her blood pressure, still enjoyed cake at birthdays. Adriana, who rebuilt her skin health, still craved fast food occasionally.

None of them lived without missteps. What mattered was persistence. What mattered was that their kitchens supported their health most of the time, not all the time.

That is the secret of prevention. It's not about rigid control. It's about creating a home, a pantry, and a rhythm of meals that make the healthy choice the natural choice.

It's about:

- Beans ready in the fridge
- Roasted vegetables on a sheet pan
- Olive oil in the cupboard
- Water on the desk
- Replacing soda with lemon water
- Replacing white bread with whole grains
- Replacing processed meat with lentils

It's about turning food into habit, not discipline.

We live in a culture that rewards speed and convenience. But look at the price: 422 million people with diabetes, 18 million deaths from heart disease each year, and rising rates of depression and dementia.

These are not genetic inevitabilities. They are the consequences of decades of processed foods, refined sugars, sedentary habits, and stress.

Prevention is the rebellion against that culture. Prevention says: my health is not for sale, my years are not disposable, my body deserves better.

Every choice matters:

- A salad at lunch lowers blood pressure that evening
- A serving of berries protects DNA that day
- A spoonful of flaxseed lowers breast cancer risk across decades
- A fish meal twice a week protects mood and memory for years

Food is not slow medicine. It is immediate and cumulative at the same time.

As a psychiatrist, I tell my patients: medication helps, therapy heals, but without food, the brain cannot recover fully.

As a physician, I tell my patients: medication lowers risk, surgery saves lives, but without food, disease keeps coming back.

As a daughter and a woman who watched her family die too young, I say: food is the difference between repeating the past and authoring a new story.

If you take one lesson from this chapter, let it be this: You are not powerless.

You can lower your risk of heart disease by thirty percent, cut your risk of diabetes in half, and triple your chance of depression remission—not with a miracle drug, but with what you put on your plate.

You can protect your skin, hair, brain, and bones not with expensive creams or procedures, but with the ordinary magic of beans, greens, olive oil, berries, and water.

The future of your health begins with prevention. The first prescription is food.

Write it every day—not in ink, but in meals you prepare, share, and savor.

And remember: the most powerful medicine may already be sitting in your kitchen.

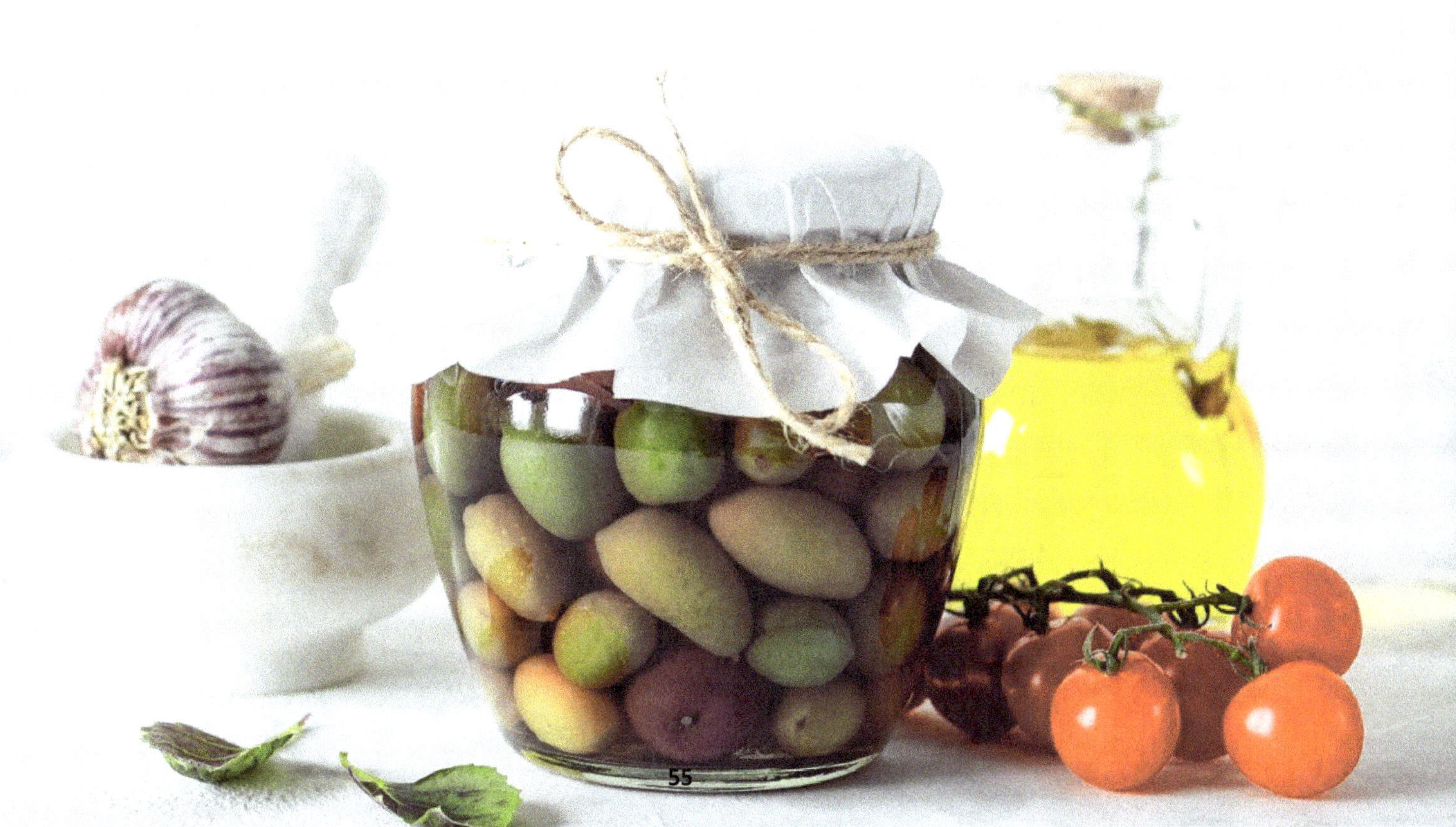

CHAPTER 3
Healing Chronic Illness & Mental Health

When Chronic Becomes Reversible

Walk into any hospital ward in the world and you will see the quiet devastation of chronic illness. A woman recovering from chemotherapy. A man with chest scarred from bypass surgery. A patient wheezing with oxygen tubing at the bedside. A young adult trembling under the grip of depression, her body drained by years of imbalance.

Chronic illness has become the defining health challenge of our century.

Yet behind these stories, one truth echoes: chronic disease rarely arrives overnight. It builds slowly, silently, relentlessly over years of daily choices. Each sugary drink stiffens arteries. Each processed meal fans inflammation. Each skipped vegetable leaves the body more vulnerable.

By the time illness announces itself with a tumor, a stroke, or a panic attack, the ground has been prepared for decades.

For too long, medicine has focused on reacting to these crises. We intervene with pills, surgeries, and procedures after disease is established. But the most powerful intervention—prevention and reversal through food—has been sitting quietly on the sidelines, available to every person, every day.

Food is not simply fuel. Food is biochemistry, information, therapy. It switches genes on and off, calms inflammation, sharpens memory, and strengthens vessels. It is both shield and weapon.

Consider the statistics:

- Cardiovascular disease claims 18 million lives annually, yet Mediterranean-style eating can lower risk by almost a third

- Diabetes affects 422 million people globally, yet lifestyle changes cut incidence by more than half
- Depression is the leading cause of disability worldwide, yet food-centered therapy triples remission rates
- Cancer—the word that brings fear into every family—is preventable in up to half of cases through diet and lifestyle

Food is not alternative medicine. It is foundational medicine. Without it, even the most advanced drugs fight uphill battles. With it, medications, therapies, and surgeries gain allies instead of enemies.

This chapter explores the research, the lived stories, and the practical strategies that prove food heals not just bodies, but lives.

PART A: PHYSICAL ILLNESS REVERSAL

Cancer and Nutrition: Fighting at the Cellular Level

Cancer cells thrive in environments of inflammation, insulin resistance, and oxidative stress. Diet can either fuel this terrain or fight against it.

The Evidence

Plant-rich diets consistently show protective effects. High fiber intake lowers risk of colorectal cancer by supporting a healthy gut microbiome that produces butyrate—a short-chain fatty acid that calms inflammation and suppresses tumor growth.

Cruciferous vegetables—broccoli, Brussels sprouts, kale—contain glucosinolates that convert into sulforaphane, a compound shown in lab studies to trigger cancer cell death and enhance detoxification enzymes.

Flaxseed, a staple in prevention diets, provides lignans—plant estrogens that balance hormones. Breast cancer recurrence rates drop significantly in women who consume flaxseed daily (Breast Cancer Research, 2017).

Green tea polyphenols, especially EGCG, slow angiogenesis—the formation of new blood vessels that tumors use to feed themselves.

Studies of survivors reinforce this: Women treated for breast cancer who consume plant-rich diets and limit alcohol live longer and relapse less often (Lancet Oncology, 2019). Prostate cancer patients adhering to Mediterranean diets show slower disease progression.

Cancer care is not only in infusion rooms. It is also in kitchens where soups simmer, greens are sautéed, and whole grains replace refined starches.

CASE STUDY: David's Colon Cancer Defense

Background: David, sixty-two, had recently completed surgery and chemotherapy for early-stage colon cancer. A retired teacher, he had always considered himself relatively healthy but began to question how much his daily habits influenced long-term health.

The Challenge: While his treatment had been successful, he worried about recurrence and wanted a practical way to support his recovery. Rather than feeling powerless after treatment ended, he decided to focus on the one area he could control every day: his diet.

The Intervention: We built a diet centered on cancer-fighting compounds:

- Daily cruciferous vegetables: Broccoli, kale, Brussels sprouts (rich in glucosinolates and sulforaphane)
- Ground flaxseed each morning mixed into yogurt or oatmeal (rich in fiber and lignans that support gut health and reduce inflammation)
- Green tea: Replaced afternoon coffee (EGCG polyphenols)
- Beans replacing red meat: 4 nights weekly (fiber, plant protein, reduced cancer-promoting compounds)
- Extra-virgin olive oil as primary cooking fat (anti-inflammatory polyphenols)
- Alcohol reduction: Wine limited to once weekly

At first, he struggled. He craved creamy comfort foods. But we experimented: roasted broccoli with garlic and olive oil, kale blended into smoothies, lentil curries with turmeric. By month three, he looked forward to his "green meals."

The Results

- **Month 6:** Month 6: Regained lean weight, fatigue lessened, energy improved
- **Year 1:** Year 1: Cancer-free, energy stronger than before treatment
- **Year 5:** Year 5: Still cancer-free, lab markers excellent

Quote: "I know food alone isn't a cure," David often tells other survivors. "But every meal is a choice. I can't control everything that happened to me, but I can control what I put on my plate."

The Science: His recovery reflects research on colorectal cancer and diet: men with higher intakes of fiber, cruciferous vegetables, and anti-inflammatory foods had lower recurrence rates and improved survival. World Cancer Research Fund estimates 30-40% of colorectal cancer recurrences can be prevented through diet.

The Lesson: David's kitchen became his pharmacy. Food didn't cure his cancer, but it shifted the odds profoundly in his favor.

Cardiovascular Disease: Arteries That Heal

If cancer is the most feared disease, heart disease is the most relentless. It remains the number one global killer, yet food is its most reliable antidote.

The Evidence

The Lifestyle Heart Trial (Ornish, 1990) followed patients who adopted plant-based diets, exercised, and practiced stress management. Within one year, coronary artery plaques regressed—arteries were opening rather than closing.

The PREDIMED trial in Spain showed Mediterranean diet with olive oil or nuts reduced heart attacks, strokes, and cardiovascular deaths by 30%. This reduction rivaled—and in some cases surpassed—common drug therapies.

Why food works:

- Olive oil (rich in monounsaturated fats and polyphenols) lowers LDL cholesterol and improves blood vessel flexibility
- Nuts provide arginine, which enhances nitric oxide production, helping vessels relax
- Fiber from beans and oats reduces cholesterol absorption in the gut
- Even simple substitutions matter replacing butter with olive oil, red meat with lentils, soda with water

A long-term study of 90,000 adults showed that just half a tablespoon of olive oil per day lowered heart disease risk by 14% (Journal of the American College of Cardiology, 2020).

Food heals arteries before stents are needed. It stabilizes rhythms before defibrillators are implanted. It lowers pressure before medications pile up.

CASE STUDY: Samuel's Heart Recovery

At sixty-one, Samuel had already survived one angina attack. His cholesterol was high, pressure uncontrolled, weight creeping upward. "I feel like my heart is a ticking bomb," he admitted.

The Challenge: Despite medications, his cardiovascular risk remained dangerously high. He lived on fast food—burgers, fries, soda. He rarely exercised. His father had died of a heart attack at sixty, and Samuel believed he was destined for the same fate.

The Intervention: Heart disease is not just genetics—it's lifestyle interacting with genes. We designed a plan he could sustain:

- Breakfast: Oatmeal topped with walnuts and berries (instead of sausage and eggs fried in butter)
- Lunch: Lentil soup with whole grain bread and olive oil (instead of fast-food burgers)
- Dinner: Grilled salmon with roasted vegetables or chickpea stews

- Treats: Two glasses of red wine weekly (instead of nightly soda)
- Exercise: Started with 15-minute daily walks, gradually increased

The Results

- **Month 3:** Lost 12 pounds, LDL cholesterol dropped 25 points
- **Month 6:** Lost 20 pounds, LDL down 40 points, triglycerides down 70 points, blood pressure down 15 mmHg
- **Year 1:** Cardiologist reduced one medication

Quote: "I thought heart disease was my family destiny. Now I know it's not written in stone."

The Science: Samuel's recovery echoed the Lyon Diet Heart Study: patients who adopted Mediterranean-style diet after heart attack had 50-70% reduction in recurrent cardiac events. The stent opened his artery, but food kept it open.

The Lesson: Heart disease did not disappear overnight, but Samuel proved what countless studies affirm: coronary artery disease can be slowed, stabilized, and in some cases partially reversed through comprehensive lifestyle change.

Lung Disease and Food: Breathing Better

The lungs may not be the first organ we associate with diet, but nutrition has profound effects on respiratory health.

The Evidence

Chronic obstructive pulmonary disease (COPD) and asthma are both worsened by inflammation and oxidative stress. Diets rich in antioxidants—berries, leafy greens, carrots, citrus—provide compounds that neutralize free radicals damaging lung tissue.

Omega-3 fatty acids from fish and seeds reduce airway inflammation.

Large population studies reveal that people who consume fruits and vegetables regularly have up to 35% lower risk of COPD. In asthma, Mediterranean diets have been linked to improved lung function and fewer exacerbations, particularly in children.

Conversely, processed foods, fried snacks, and sugary drinks accelerate inflammation, worsen lung function, and increase risk of flareups.

In other words, food helps people breathe.

CASE STUDY: Rosa's COPD Support

Rosa, seventy, struggled with chronic obstructive pulmonary disease. Even climbing stairs left her breathless. Inhalers gave partial relief, but she wanted more. She was a lifelong smoker (quit 10 years prior) who had lived on fried foods and processed meats.

The Challenge: COPD is not reversible, but nutrition can slow progression and improve quality of life.

The Intervention: We introduced antioxidants and omega-3s:

- Daily green smoothies: Spinach, banana, berries (vitamin C, carot-enoids)
- Roasted vegetables: Instead of fried snacks (antioxidants without pro-inflammatory oils)
- Sardines twice weekly: (omega-3s, vitamin D)
- Citrus fruits daily: (vitamin C for immune support)
- Eliminated: Processed meats (linked to worse COPD outcomes)

The Results

- **Month 3:** Fewer flareups, slightly better stamina
- **Month 6:** Could climb one flight of stairs without stopping
- **Year 1:** Lung function tests stable (not declining)

Quote: "I still have COPD, but I don't feel like it owns me anymore."

The Science: Rosa's improvement reflects evidence that fruits, vegetables, and omega-3s improve lung function and reduce COPD risk (European Respiratory Journal, 2018). While food cannot reverse structural lung damage, it reduces systemic inflammation that worsens symptoms.

The Lesson: Food gave Rosa more breath—and with it, more life.

PART B: PSYCHIATRY & NUTRITION

Depression: Food as an Antidepressant Adjunct

Depression is the leading cause of disability worldwide, affecting more than 280 million people (WHO). Standard treatments include medication and therapy, both lifesavings. But not all patients respond fully. Here, diet becomes an essential, evidence-based adjunct.

The SMILES Trial

Published in BMC Medicine (2017), this was the first randomized controlled trial to test diet as a treatment for depression. Participants with major depressive disorder were assigned either a Mediterranean-style diet or social support.

After 12 weeks, 32% of the diet group achieved remission, compared to just 8% in the control group.

The diet emphasized:

- Whole grains, legumes, nuts
- Vegetables, fruit, fish, olive oil
- Reduced sweets, refined grains, processed meats, fried foods

The improvements were independent of weight loss, showing that the brain responds to nutrient composition, not just calories.

Why Diet Matters in Depression

- Inflammation: Depressed patients often have elevated inflammatory markers (CRP, IL-6). Anti-inflammatory diets reduce these.
- Neuroplasticity: Nutrients like omega-3s, folate, zinc, and polyphenols increase brain-derived neurotrophic factor (BDNF), which supports synapse growth.
- Neurotransmitter synthesis: Amino acids (tryptophan, tyrosine) and B-vitamins are precursors for serotonin, dopamine, and norepinephrine.
- Microbiome: A healthy gut microbiota produces short-chain fatty acids and serotonin precursors, directly communicating with the brain via the vagus nerve.

CASE STUDY: Elena's Depression Recovery

Elena, forty, was a nurse who had battled depression for years. Medications dulled her symptoms but left her fatigued. She often skipped meals and relied on pastries and coffee to keep going during shifts.

The Challenge: Her antidepressants helped, but she felt only partially recovered—still flat, still exhausted, still disconnected from joy.

The Intervention: We rebuilt her diet from the ground up:

- Breakfast: Oats with walnuts and blueberries (stable glucose, omega-3s, polyphenols)
- Lunch: Lentil salad with olive oil and greens (protein, fiber, folate, magnesium)
- Dinner: Salmon with roasted vegetables (DHA omega-3s, vitamin D, antioxidants)

Added: Fermented foods like kefir and sauerkraut (probiotics for gut-brain axis)

Eliminated: Skipping meals, relying on sugar for energy

The Results

- **Month 1:** Sleep improved (fewer middle-of-night wakings)
- **Month 2:** Energy increased, fewer crying spells
- **Month 3:** Mood described as "lighter," PHQ-9 depression score dropped by half

- **Month 6:** Psychiatrist noted antidepressant worked more effectively when paired with dietary change

Quote: "Food didn't cure my depression, but it gave my medication something to work with. I finally feel like myself again."

The Science: Elena's recovery mirrors research showing food doesn't replace therapy or medication but potentiates them. Her story echoes Harvard findings: plant-based diets reduce depression risk by 25%.

The Lesson: Food nourishes not only the body but the brain. When nutrition fails, even the best medications struggle. When nutrition succeeds, recovery accelerates.

Anxiety: Stabilizing a Restless Mind

Anxiety disorders affect 1 in 5 adults in the United States. They are characterized by hyperarousal of the nervous system—racing thoughts, pounding heart, shallow breathing. While therapy and medication remain crucial, nutrition often plays an invisible role.

Blood Sugar and Adrenaline

Sharp spikes and crashes in blood glucose trigger adrenaline release. Patients describe this as "feeling like a panic attack." Diets high in refined carbs and sugar exacerbate these swings.

In contrast, protein-rich, fiber-rich meals stabilize glucose and reduce physiological triggers of anxiety.

Omega-3 Fatty Acids

Meta-analyses show that omega-3 supplementation (particularly EPA) reduces anxiety symptoms (Frontiers in Psychiatry, 2020). Mechanisms include dampening of inflammation and stabilization of neuronal membranes.

Magnesium

Found in leafy greens, nuts, legumes, and seeds, magnesium calms the nervous system by regulating neurotransmitters and reducing cortisol.

CASE STUDY: Hannah's Anxiety Calm

Hannah, thirty-six, was a mother with generalized anxiety disorder. She skipped breakfast, lived on coffee, and snacked on pastries. Her evenings ended with pasta and wine. She described feeling "wired but tired."

The Challenge: Her anxiety was constant—racing heart, tight chest, restless nights. Medication helped partially, but she still felt on edge.

The Intervention: We focused on stabilizing glucose and calming the nervous system:

- Breakfast: Smoothie with kefir, flaxseed, banana, spinach (probiotics, omega-3 precursors, magnesium)
- Lunch: Black beans, avocado, brown rice (protein, fiber, potassium, steady energy)
- Dinner: Salmon and vegetables (omega-3s, magnesium from greens)
- Coffee: Cut after noon, replaced with green tea (L-theanine smooths cortisol response)

Added: Magnesium-rich foods daily (spinach, pumpkin seeds, almonds)

The Results

- **Week 2:** Sleep deeper, fewer middle-of-night anxiety spikes
- **Month 1:** Panic attacks decreased from 5/week to 1/week
- **Month 3:** Baseline tension lower, therapy more effective

Quote: "My anxiety didn't disappear, but my body stopped amplifying it.

I finally feel like I can breathe."

The Science: Hannah's improvement reflects Nutrients (2019): dietary interventions reduced anxiety scores by 25-30%. Stable glucose prevents adrenaline surges, omega-3s calm inflammation, magnesium regulates stress response.

The Lesson: Nutrition lowered Hannah's physiological "alarm system," allowing therapy and medication to reach deeper.

ADHD: Fueling Focus

ADHD affects both children and adults. While stimulant medication is often effective, diet can shape symptoms dramatically.

The Role of Sugar and Additives

High sugar intake exacerbates hyperactivity. Artificial dyes and preservatives have been linked in multiple studies to worsened symptoms, particularly in children.

Omega-3 Evidence

A meta-analysis in European Neuropsychopharmacology (2017) found that omega-3 supplementation improves attention and reduces hyperactivity in ADHD. The effect is modest but meaningful, especially in patients with low baseline omega-3 intake.

Protein and Iron

Protein-rich breakfasts improve focus by stabilizing blood sugar and providing amino acids for dopamine synthesis. Iron deficiency can mimic or worsen ADHD symptoms.

CASE STUDY: My ADHD Journey & Jamal's Breakthrough

My Story

During my decisive step of medical licensure, I faced ADHD head-on. After failing the exam five times, I sought help. With the right medication combined with:

- Hydration (dehydration worsens attention)
- Structured nutrition (high-protein breakfasts, reduced sugar, consistent meals)
- Exercise (daily movement improves executive function)

I found the focus I needed. On my final attempt, I passed.

If I had not combined medication with lifestyle, I would not be a physician in the United States today. It was a victory fueled by food, movement, and resilience.

Jamal's Story

Jamal, twenty-two, was a college student who had failed two classes despite taking medication. His diet revolved around energy drinks and late-night fast food.

The Intervention:

- Protein-rich breakfasts: Eggs and spinach (dopamine precursors)
- Omega-3 supplementation: Fish oil + salmon 2x/week
- Eliminated energy drinks: Replaced with water and green tea
- Vegetables with every meal: Magnesium, iron, B-vitamins

The Results:

- **Month 3:** Focus during lectures improved dramatically Semester end: Passed his exams

Quote: "If I hadn't changed my food, medication alone wouldn't have been enough."

The Science: Our experiences reflect research: omega-3s, protein, iron, and stable glucose improve ADHD symptoms (Nutrients, 2020). Food doesn't replace medication—it makes medication work better.

The Lesson: ADHD is not a life sentence of struggle. With the right combination of medication, nutrition, and structure, focus returns.

Bipolar Disorder: Food for Stability

Bipolar disorder is a lifelong condition marked by swings between mania and depression. While medication is essential, diet can support stability.

Omega-3 Studies

In a landmark trial published in Archives of General Psychiatry, patients with bipolar disorder given omega-3 supplements had longer periods of remission compared to placebo.

Glycemic Control

Erratic eating patterns and high-sugar diets worsen mood swings by destabilizing glucose and sleep. Structured meals with complex carbohydrates and protein reduce volatility.

CASE STUDY: Michael's Bipolar Balance

Michael, forty, was a graphic designer with bipolar II disorder. His diet was chaotic—sometimes fasting until dinner, then overeating sugary foods. His mood mirrored his meals: unstable, crashing after binges, restless during long gaps.

The Challenge: Despite medication, his depressive episodes still stole months of his life. He felt powerless over his body.

The Intervention: We introduced rhythm and nutrition:

- Three structured meals daily: Each with complex carbs, protein, healthy fats
- Leafy greens, beans, salmon, walnuts: Daily staples (magnesium, omega-3s, B-vitamins)
- Reduced alcohol: No more than 2 drinks/week

Eliminated: Late-night snacking (replaced with herbal tea)

The Results

- **Month 3:** Depressive episodes shorter
- **Month 6:** Psychiatrist adjusted medications less often Year 1: Mood more stable, energy steadier

Quote: "I finally feel like my body and mind are aligned. Food gave me guardrails."

The Science: Michael's stability reflects research: omega-3s reduce depressive relapses in bipolar disorder (Journal of Clinical Psychiatry, 2016). Structured meals prevent glucose-driven mood swings.

The Lesson: Food doesn't cure bipolar disorder, but it provides the foundation for medications and therapy to work.

Trauma Recovery: Calming the Alarm System

Post-traumatic stress disorder (PTSD) and trauma-related disorders are not only psychological—they are physiological states of chronic hyperarousal. Elevated cortisol, heightened inflammation, and disturbed sleep make trauma recovery not just emotional but biological.

The Evidence

Anti-inflammatory diets help regulate stress hormones, reduce inflammatory signaling, and support sleep (Frontiers in Psychology, 2020).

Diets rich in:

- Omega-3s (reduce cortisol surges)
- Magnesium (calms nervous system)
- Probiotics (restore gut health disrupted by chronic stress)

...have been shown to reduce PTSD severity.

CASE STUDY: Sofia's Nightmares Fade

Sofia, thirty-two, was a teacher who carried scars of childhood abuse. She had nightmares, flashbacks, and a constant sense of danger. Therapy and medication helped, but she still felt "wired for fear."

The Challenge: Her diet was filled with processed foods and sugary snacks—patterns developed as coping mechanisms during trauma.

The Intervention: We rebuilt her plate with anti-inflammatory nutrients:

- Salmon twice weekly: (omega-3s reduce cortisol and inflammation)
- Walnuts and flaxseed daily: (plant omega-3 precursors)
- Leafy greens and blueberries: (antioxidants calm oxidative stress)
- Reduced sugar and refined carbs: (stabilize mood, prevent crashes)
- Added chamomile tea: (calming ritual before bed)

The Results

- **Month 1:** Sleep improved (fewer middle-of-night wakings)
- **Month 3:** Nightmares less frequent (from nightly to 1-2x/week)
- **Month 6:** Panic surges decreased during the day

Quote: "Food didn't erase my trauma, but it lowered my body's alarm. I can finally rest."

The Science: Sofia's recovery reflects Frontiers in Psychiatry (2019): patients with higher intakes of omega-3s and antioxidants had reduced PTSD severity.

The Lesson: For trauma survivors, food is not a cure—but it calms the physiological storm, allowing therapy to work more effectively.

OCD: Nutrition as a Stabilizer

Obsessive-compulsive disorder is driven by anxiety and intrusive thoughts that push people into repetitive behaviors. While medication and therapy are first-line treatments, nutrition influences the body's stress baseline.

The Evidence

Magnesium and zinc regulate neurotransmitters involved in anxiety. Stable glucose prevents adrenaline surges that intensify intrusive thoughts. Omega-3s improve communication between brain regions involved in impulse control.

CASE STUDY: Daniel's Compulsions Quieted

Daniel, twenty-four, battled compulsions that consumed his evenings (4+ hours of rituals). His diet was dominated by fast food and caffeine.

The Challenge: Despite medication and therapy, his compulsions remained overwhelming.

The Intervention: We shifted his meals to stabilize neurotransmitter precursors:

- Oatmeal with walnuts (breakfast for stable energy)
- Salmon twice weekly: (omega-3s for brain communication)
- Spinach-based salads daily: (magnesium, folate)
- Cut caffeine after noon: (reduced anxiety spikes)
- Added magnesium-rich foods: Beans, pumpkin seeds

The Results

- **Month 2:** Compulsions reduced from 4 hours to 2 hours daily
- **Month 4:** Anxiety baseline lower, therapy more effective

Quote: "My urges are still there, but they're quieter. I don't feel controlled anymore."

The Science: Daniel's improvement reflects Journal of Psychiatric Research (2016): omega-3 fatty acids and magnesium can modulate anxiety-related symptoms, making OCD treatment more effective.

The Lesson: Nutrition doesn't eliminate OCD, but it reduces the physiological noise that amplifies compulsions.

Developmental Disorders: The Gut-Brain Axis

Autism spectrum disorder and ADHD highlight the importance of nutrition in developmental conditions. The gut-brain axis—communication between intestinal microbes and the nervous system—is now recognized as a key player.

Children with autism often experience gastrointestinal symptoms, picky eating, and nutrient deficiencies. Diet adjustments that focus on omega-3s, probiotics, and elimination of artificial dyes can improve behavior and focus.

CASE STUDY: Lila's Transformation

Lila, seven, had autism spectrum disorder. Her parents were exhausted—worried about her tantrums, limited diet (crackers, milk, sweets), and constant gastrointestinal discomfort.

The Challenge: She ate almost no vegetables, refused most proteins, and her gut health was clearly compromised (frequent constipation, bloating).

The Intervention: We slowly introduced new foods:

- Berries blended into smoothies: (antioxidants, palatability)
- Spinach hidden in pasta sauce: (folate, iron)
- Flaxseed stirred into yogurt: (omega-3 precursors)
- Probiotics through kefir: (gut-brain support)
- Eliminated artificial dyes: (linked to behavioral issues)

The Results

- **Month 3:** Digestion improved (less constipation, less bloating)
- **Month 6:** Fewer tantrums, calmer evenings, teachers noted better focus
- **Year 1:** Quality of life significantly improved

Quote (from parents): "Her autism didn't disappear, but she's calmer, happier, more present."

The Science: Lila's improvements reflect Frontiers in Pediatrics (2020): improving gut health reduces irritability and supports better attention in children with autism.

The Lesson: Food cannot cure developmental disorders, but it can ease suffering and improve function—giving children and families a better quality of life.

PART C: THE PSYCHOLOGY OF EATING

Emotional Eating: Comfort or Cage?

Emotional eating is the tendency to use food for comfort, stress relief, or reward. While occasional indulgence is normal, chronic emotional eating becomes a cycle of guilt, shame, and worsening health.

The Evidence

A study in Appetite (2013) found that stress increases preference for high-sugar, high-fat foods.

The American Psychological Association (APA) Stress in America Report shows that 38% of adults report overeating or eating unhealthy foods because of stress at least once per week.

High-sugar comfort foods trigger dopamine release in the brain's reward center, temporarily soothing but reinforcing cravings.

CASE STUDY: Laura's Late-Night Eating

Laura, thirty-five, was a teacher struggling with weight gain and anxiety. Every evening, after her children were asleep, she ate ice cream and chips to "relax." She said it was the only time she felt she could reward herself.

The Challenge: Food had become her only coping mechanism for stress. She felt trapped in a cycle of guilt and shame.

The Intervention: We reframed her strategy:

- Replaced late-night sugar with: Chamomile tea and fruit
- Added stress release: 20-minute evening walks
- Journaling emotions: Instead of eating them
- Mindful eating practice: Paying attention to hunger vs. emotion

The Results

- **Month 3:** Lost 10 pounds, sleep improved
- **Month 6:** Lost 15 pounds, anxiety "finally manageable"

Quote: "I realized I wasn't hungry—I was exhausted and overwhelmed. Now I have tools besides food."

The Science: Laura's story reflects research showing emotional eating is a learned coping mechanism that can be unlearned and replaced with healthier practices.

The Lesson: Food is not the enemy—but using it to numb emotions creates more suffering. When we address the underlying emotions, food returns to its proper role: nourishment.

Food Addiction: When Cravings Control the Brain

Food addiction is increasingly recognized as a behavioral and neurological disorder. It shares mechanisms with substance addiction: dopamine surges, tolerance, and withdrawal.

The Evidence

The Yale Food Addiction Scale estimates that 5-10% of the population meets criteria for food addiction, with higher rates in obesity.

Neuroimaging studies show that sugar activates the same brain reward pathways as cocaine and opioids.

In Frontiers in Psychiatry (2018), researchers concluded that "highly processed foods with added fats and refined carbohydrates are most implicated in addictive-like eating behaviors."

CASE STUDY: Ethan's Sugar Battle

Ethan, forty, described himself as a "sugar addict." He ate candy at his desk, drank multiple sodas daily, and panicked if he ran out. His attempts to "cut back" led to headaches, irritability, and cravings—classic withdrawal symptoms.

The Challenge: He felt controlled by sugar. Every attempt to quit ended in failure.

The Intervention: We treated it like an addiction:

- Gradual reduction: Not cold turkey (to avoid overwhelming withdrawal)
- Replaced soda: With sparkling water, then gradually plain water
- Increased protein and fiber: To stabilize blood sugar and reduce cravings
- Addressed triggers: Stress at work led to candy → replaced with nuts and water

The Results

- **Month 1:** Headaches subsided, cravings decreased
- **Month 3:** Lost 10 pounds, cravings "almost gone"
- **Month 6:** No longer felt controlled by sugar

Quote: "I didn't think I could break free. Now I realize sugar had hijacked my brain—but I took it back."

The Science: Ethan's recovery reinforces the concept that food addiction is real, measurable, and treatable with structured strategies.

The Lesson: Sugar is not simply "willpower"—it's brain chemistry. When we treat it as an addiction, recovery becomes possible.

Body Image and Identity: Eating with Purpose

Food is tied to identity. Cultural traditions, family patterns, and personal values shape choices. Unfortunately, body image pressures often distort these relationships, leading to restrictive diets or binge patterns.

The Statistics

According to the National Alliance for Eating Disorders (NAED), 20 million women and 10 million men in the U.S. will experience an eating disorder in their lifetime.

Diet culture, driven by media, contributes to unhealthy cycles of restriction and bingeing.

Plant-rich, Mediterranean, and Blue Zones-style eating patterns not only improve health outcomes but also foster sustainable, positive relationships with food.

CASE STUDY: Jasmine's Body Image Healing

Jasmine, twenty-eight, was an artist who cycled between restrictive dieting and bingeing. She described hating her body and fearing food.

The Challenge: Her relationship with food was punishment, not nourishment.

The Intervention: We shifted her goal from "being thin" to "being strong and healthy":

- Mediterranean-style meals: Beans, greens, olive oil, fish
- Exercise for energy: Not weight loss (Pilates, walking)
- Therapy: To address body image distortions
- Mindful eating: To reconnect with hunger and fullness cues

The Results

- **Month 3:** Bingeing episodes decreased
- **Month 6:** Improved mood, reduced restriction Year 1: Newfound confidence

Quote: "Food is no longer my enemy. It's my fuel, my pleasure, my partner."

The Science: Jasmine's recovery reflects International Journal of Eating Disorders (2019): combined cognitive-behavioral therapy (CBT) and nutritional counseling produced better recovery outcomes than therapy alone.

The Lesson: When we reframe food as nourishment rather than punishment, healing begins.

SECTION 3: TOOLKIT FOR HEALING

Shopping List Essentials

Pantry Staples:

- Beans and lentils (canned and dry)
- Whole grains: oats, quinoa, barley, brown rice
- Nuts and seeds: walnuts, almonds, chia, flax, pumpkin seeds

- Extra virgin olive oil
- Canned tomatoes, vegetable broth

Refrigerator:

- Leafy greens: spinach, kale, arugula
- Cruciferous vegetables: broccoli, cauliflower, Brussels sprouts
- Berries (fresh or frozen)
- Fermented foods: kefir, yogurt, sauerkraut
- Eggs

Freezer:

- Salmon, sardines (or canned in pantry)
- Frozen vegetables
- Frozen berries

Quick Swaps for Healing

Instead of...	Try this...
Processed breakfast cereal	Oatmeal with berries and walnuts
Fast food lunch	Lentil soup with whole grain bread
Fried snacks	Roasted chickpeas or nuts
Sugary desserts	Dark chocolate + fruit
Energy drinks	Green tea + water
White pasta	Whole grain pasta or lentil pasta

Food Prescriptions by Condition

- Cancer: Cruciferous vegetables, flaxseed, green tea, beans, berries
- Heart Disease: Oats, beans, olive oil, walnuts, salmon
- Lung Disease: Berries, citrus, omega-3s, leafy greens
- Depression: Salmon, walnuts, probiotics (kefir), leafy greens
- Anxiety: Magnesium-rich foods (spinach, pumpkin seeds), omega-3s, green tea
- ADHD: Protein-rich breakfasts, omega-3s, iron-rich foods (lentils, spinach)
- Bipolar: Structured meals, omega-3s, complex carbs
- Trauma/PTSD: Anti-inflammatory foods (salmon, berries, leafy greens, olive oil)
- OCD: Magnesium, zinc, omega-3s, stable glucose
- Emotional Eating: Fiber-rich meals, protein, mindful eating practices

SECTION 4: 7-DAY HEALING MEAL PLAN

GOAL: Support healing across physical illness, mental health, and emotional well-being
FOCUS: Anti-inflammatory compounds, stable glucose, omega-3s, probiotics, antioxidants

DAY 1: FOUNDATION

MORNING Overnight Oats with Chia & Walnuts: Oats + chia + blue-berries + walnuts. **Why:** Fiber + omega-3s + polyphenols = stable mood, reduced inflammation

MIDDAY Turmeric Lentil Soup: Lentils + spinach + turmeric + olive oil. **Why:** Curcumin calms inflammation, magnesium supports nervous system

EVENING Salmon with Quinoa & Broccoli: DHA omega-3s + complete protein + sulforaphane. **Why:** Brain repair, cancer protection, cardiovascular support

DAILY PRACTICE: Walk 15 minutes, journal emotions

DAY 2: STABILITY

MORNING Greek Yogurt Probiotic Bowl: Yogurt + raspberries + almonds + cinnamon. **Why:** Probiotics support gut-brain axis, berries reduce oxidative stress

MIDDAY Chickpea Salad: Chickpeas + cucumber + tomatoes + parsley + olive oil.

Why: Resistant starch feeds gut bacteria, steady energy

EVENING Cod with Kale & Sweet Potato: Lean protein + magnesium + beta-carotene. **Why:** Supports dopamine production, reduces inflammation

DAILY PRACTICE: Replace coffee after noon with green tea

DAY 3: MENTAL CLARITY

MORNING Eggs with Spinach & Sourdough: Choline + folate + slow digesting.
Why : Improves memory, lowers depression risk, steady focus

MIDDAY Black Bean Bowl: Black beans + avocado + lime + brown rice.

Why: Magnesium calms anxiety, potassium lowers blood pressure

EVENING Mediterranean Vegetable Bake: Eggplant + zucchini + peppers + barley.

Why: Antioxidant spectrum, cholesterol reduction

DAILY PRACTICE: 5 minutes mindful eating

DAY 4: GUT-BRAIN HEALING

MORNING Probiotic Smoothie: Kefir + banana + spinach + pumpkin seeds + green tea. **Why:** Probiotics + prebiotic fiber + L-theanine = calm focus

MIDDAY Sardinian Minestrone: Beans + barley + kale + rosemary.
Why: Longevity staple, fiber, plant protein

EVENING Sardines on Toast: Whole grain + sardines + tomatoes + carrots.
Why: Omega-3s + vitamin D + calcium + lycopene

DAILY PRACTICE: Journal how you feel after each meal

DAY 5: ANTI-INFLAMMATORY

MORNING Flax Oatmeal: Oatmeal + flaxseed + apple + cinnamon.

Why: Lignans + quercetin = cancer protection, inflammation reduction

MIDDAY Hummus Plate: Hummus + vegetables + olives + whole grain pita.
Why: Polyphenols, stable glucose, calcium

EVENING Roasted Chicken with Lentils: Chicken + arugula salad + lentils.
Why: Nitrates improve vascular health, folate supports mood

DAILY PRACTICE: Dark chocolate (70%+) instead of pastries

DAY 6: STRENGTH & RECOVERY

MORNING Kefir Berry Bowl: Kefir + blueberries + chia.
Why: Probiotics repair gut, antioxidants protect neurons

MIDDAY Chickpea Turmeric Stew: Chickpeas + spinach + turmeric.

Why: Curcumin + iron + fiber = healing trifecta

EVENING Grilled Salmon with Quinoa & Peppers: Omega-3s + complete protein + vitamin C.
Why: Athletic recovery, mood support, cardio-vascular protection

DAILY PRACTICE: 20 minutes resistance training

DAY 7: INTEGRATION

MORNING Chia Pudding: Chia + almond milk + pomegranate + walnuts (prepared night before). **Why:** Punicalagins reduce vascular inflammation, omega-3s support brain

MIDDAY Probiotic Veggie Wrap: Whole grain wrap + avocado + black beans + sauerkraut.
Why: Complete gut-brain meal

EVENING Mediterranean Grain Bowl: Quinoa + chickpeas + vegetables + herbs + olive oil.
Why: Prevention bowl—cardiovascular + cancer protection

DAILY PRACTICE: Write three changes noticed this week

SECTION 5: SEVEN HEALING RECIPES

1. ANTI-INFLAMMATORY GOLDEN LENTILS (Featured Recipe)

Curcumin-powered comfort that calms the body from within.

SERVES: 6 | **PREP:** 10 min | **COOK:** 35 min

WHY IT WORKS *This dish combines cholesterol-lowering lentils with turmeric's anti-inflammatory curcumin. Perfect for managing arthritis, heart disease, depression, or chronic inflammation. It is comfort food that heals.*

INGREDIENTS

For the base:

- 2 tablespoons coconut oil or olive oil
- 1 onion, diced
- 3 garlic cloves, minced
- 1 tablespoon fresh ginger, grated

For the lentils:

- 1 cup red lentils, rinsed
- 1 can (14 oz) coconut milk
- 2 cups vegetable broth
- 2 teaspoons ground turmeric
- 1 teaspoon ground cumin
- ½ teaspoon black pepper (activates curcumin)
- 1 teaspoon salt

To finish:

- 2 cups fresh spinach
- Juice of 1 lime
- Fresh cilantro, chopped

METHOD

1. Heat oil in a large pot over medium heat. Sauté onion until softened (5 minutes).
2. Add garlic and ginger, stir for 1 minute until fragrant.
3. Add turmeric, cumin, and black pepper. Stir for 30 seconds.
4. Add lentils, coconut milk, and broth. Bring to a boil.
5. Reduce heat and simmer for 20-25 minutes until lentils are soft.
6. Stir in spinach until wilted.
7. Remove from heat, add lime juice.
8. Serve over brown rice or quinoa, garnished with fresh cilantro.

THE SCIENCE Turmeric's curcumin reduces inflammatory markers like CRP and IL-6 (Journal of Medicinal Food, 2016). Black pepper increases curcumin absorption by 2,000%. Lentils stabilize blood sugar and lower cholesterol. Coconut milk adds medium-chain triglycerides (MCTs) that support brain health.

NUTRITIONAL HIGHLIGHTS ~280 calories per serving | Rich in: Fiber (8g), Protein (10g), Curcumin, Iron

VARIATIONS

- Extra vegetables: Add diced sweet potato or carrots
- Spicier: Add cayenne or red chili flakes
- Depression support: Serve with salmon on the side (omega-3 boost)

STORAGE Refrigerate up to 5 days. Freezes well for 3 months.

2. CANCER-FIGHTING BROCCOLI FLAXSEED SALAD (Featured Recipe)

Cruciferous power meets hormone-balancing lignans.

SERVES: 4 | **PREP:** 10 min | **COOK:** 5 min

WHY IT WORKS *This salad delivers sulforaphane from broccoli (activates detoxification enzymes) and lignans from flaxseed (modulates estrogen). Perfect for cancer survivors and those focused on prevention.*

INGREDIENTS

For the salad:

- 4 cups broccoli florets
- 2 cups baby spinach or arugula
- ¼ cup red onion, thinly sliced
- ¼ cup pomegranate seeds

For the dressing:

- 3 tablespoons extra virgin olive oil
- Juice of 1 lemon
- 2 tablespoons ground flaxseed
- 1 garlic clove, minced
- Salt and pepper to taste

METHOD

1. Steam broccoli for 3-4 minutes until bright green and tender-crisp. Cool under chilly water.
2. In a large bowl, combine broccoli, spinach, red onion, and pomegranate seeds.
3. In a small bowl, whisk together olive oil, lemon juice, ground flax-seed, garlic, salt, and pepper.
4. Pour dressing over salad and toss gently.
5. Let sit for 10 minutes to allow flax to soften and flavors to meld.

THE SCIENCE Broccoli's sulforaphane triggers phase II detoxification enzymes that neutralize carcinogens (Cancer Prevention Research, 2015). Flaxseed lignans modulate estrogen metabolism and reduce breast cancer risk (Breast Cancer Research, 2017). Pomegranate adds punicalagins for cardiovascular protection.

NUTRITIONAL HIGHLIGHTS ~180 calories per serving | Rich in: Fiber (7g), Sulforaphane, Lignans, Vitamin C

VARIATIONS

- Extra protein: Top with grilled chicken or chickpeas
- Nut version: Add chopped walnuts for omega-3s
- Make ahead: Prepare components separately, dress just before serving

STORAGE Best fresh. Components can be prepped ahead and assembled same day.

3. HEART-HEALING OAT & WALNUT BOWL (Featured Recipe)

Cholesterol-lowering fiber meets brain-boosting omega-3s.

SERVES: 2 | **PREP:** 5 min | **COOK:** 10 min

WHY IT WORKS *This breakfast bowl combines soluble fiber from oats (proven to lower LDL cholesterol) with omega-3s from walnuts and antioxidants from blueberries. Perfect for cardiovascular protection and cognitive support.*

INGREDIENTS

- 1 cup rolled oats
- 2 cups water or almond milk
- Pinch of salt
- 1 teaspoon cinnamon
- ½ cup fresh or frozen blueberries
- ¼ cup chopped walnuts
- 1 tablespoon ground flaxseed
- Optional: 1 teaspoon honey or maple syrup

METHOD

1. In a small pot, bring water or milk to a boil.
2. Add oats, salt, and cinnamon. Reduce heat to low.
3. Simmer for 5-7 minutes, stirring occasionally, until creamy.
4. Remove from heat. Divide between two bowls.
5. Top each bowl with blueberries, walnuts, and flaxseed.
6. Drizzle with honey if desired.

THE SCIENCE Oats contain beta-glucan, a soluble fiber that lowers LDL cholesterol by 5-10% (American Journal of Clinical Nutrition, 2014). Walnuts provide alpha-linolenic acid (plant omega-3) that reduces cardiovascular mortality (Circulation, 2018). Blueberries' anthocyanins protect DNA and improve memory (Nutrients, 2020).

NUTRITIONAL HIGHLIGHTS ~320 calories per serving | Rich in: Fiber (10g), Omega-3s, Polyphenols, Magnesium

VARIATIONS

- Extra protein: Stir in Greek yogurt
- Savory version: Skip sweet toppings, add chia seeds and a drizzle of olive oil
- Make ahead: Overnight oats version (mix oats with milk, refrigerate, add toppings in morning)

STORAGE Best fresh. Overnight version lasts 3 days refrigerated.

4. ADHD-FOCUS SALMON BAKE (Featured Recipe)

Protein + omega-3s + iron = sustained attention.

SERVES: 4 | **PREP:** 10 min | **COOK:** 20 min

WHY IT WORKS *This one-pan meal combines DHA omega-3s from salmon (improves neurotransmitter signaling), iron and folate from spinach (prevents attention deficits), and complex carbs from sweet potatoes (stable glucose = stable focus).*

INGREDIENTS

For the salmon:

- 4 salmon fillets (4-6 oz each)
- 2 tablespoons olive oil
- 1 lemon, sliced
- Salt and pepper

For the vegetables:

- 2 large sweet potatoes, cubed
- 4 cups fresh spinach
- 2 garlic cloves, minced
- 1 tablespoon olive oil
- ½ teaspoon paprika

METHOD

1. Preheat oven to 400°F (200°C).
2. Toss sweet potato cubes with 1 tablespoon olive oil, paprika, salt, and pepper. Spread on one side of a large baking sheet.
3. Place salmon fillets on the other side. Brush with remaining olive oil, top with lemon slices, season with salt and pepper.
4. Bake for 15-18 minutes until salmon flakes easily and sweet potatoes are tender.
5. Meanwhile, sauté spinach with garlic in a skillet until wilted (2 minutes).
6. Serve salmon and sweet potatoes over sautéed spinach.

THE SCIENCE DHA omega-3s improve attention and reduce hyperactivity in ADHD (Nutrients, 2020). Iron deficiency can mimic ADHD symptoms; spinach provides bioavailable iron. Sweet potatoes offer sustained glucose release, preventing attention crashes.

NUTRITIONAL HIGHLIGHTS ~420 calories per serving | Rich in: Omega-3s (2g), Protein (32g), Iron, Beta-carotene

VARIATIONS

- Budget version: Use sardines instead of salmon
- Extra iron: Add lentils on the side
- Kid-friendly: Mash sweet potatoes, blend spinach into a sauce

STORAGE Refrigerate up to 3 days. Reheat gently in oven.

5. DEPRESSION-LIFTING MEDITERRANEAN BOWL (Featured Recipe)

Serotonin support in every bite.

SERVES: 4 | **PREP:** 15 min (if grains pre-cooked) | **COOK:** 0 min

WHY IT WORKS *This bowl mirrors the SMILES Trial diet that tripled depression remission rates. It combines tryptophan-rich chickpeas, omega-3-rich walnuts, folate-rich greens, and polyphenol-rich olive oil—all nutrients that support neurotransmitter synthesis and reduce inflammation.*

INGREDIENTS

For the base:

- 2 cups cooked quinoa or brown rice
- 1 can (15 oz) chickpeas, drained
- 3 cups mixed greens (spinach, arugula, romaine)

For the bowl:

- 1 cup cherry tomatoes, halved
- 1 cucumber, diced
- ¼ cup Kalamata olives
- ¼ cup chopped walnuts
- ¼ cup crumbled feta (optional)

For the dressing:

- 3 tablespoons extra virgin olive oil
- Juice of 1 lemon
- 1 tablespoon tahini
- 1 garlic clove, minced
- 1 teaspoon dried oregano
- Salt and pepper

METHOD

1. In a large bowl, combine quinoa, chickpeas, and mixed greens.
2. Add tomatoes, cucumber, olives, and walnuts.
3. In a small bowl, whisk together olive oil, lemon juice, tahini, garlic, oregano, salt, and pepper.
4. Pour dressing over bowl and toss gently.
5. Top with feta if using.
6. Serve at room temperature or chilled.

THE SCIENCE This combination mirrors the SMILES Trial (BMC Medicine, 2017): Mediterranean diet improved depression remission by 32%. Chickpeas provide tryptophan (serotonin precursor), walnuts provide omega-3s (improve neurotransmitter signaling), greens provide folate (deficiency linked to depression), olive oil reduces neuroinflammation.

NUTRITIONAL HIGHLIGHTS ~450 calories per serving | Rich in: Fiber (12g), Protein (14g), Omega-3s, Folate

VARIATIONS

- Extra protein: Add grilled chicken or tofu
- Warm version: Heat quinoa and chickpeas before assembling
- Simpler: Use store-bought tahini dressing

STORAGE Components can be prepped ahead. Dress just before serving. Lasts 3 days refrigerated.

6. TRAUMA-RECOVERY ANTI-INFLAMMATORY STEW (Featured Recipe)

Calming the body's alarm system, one bowl at a time.

SERVES: 6 | **PREP:** 15 min | **COOK:** 40 min

WHY IT WORKS *This stew is designed to reduce cortisol and inflam-mation—both elevated in trauma survivors. It combines omega-3-rich fish, curcumin from turmeric, and magnesium from greens to calm the nervous system and support resilience.*

INGREDIENTS

For the base:

- 2 tablespoons olive oil
- 1 onion, diced
- 3 garlic cloves, minced
- 1 tablespoon fresh ginger, grated
- 1 tablespoon ground turmeric
- 1 teaspoon ground cumin
- ½ teaspoon black pepper

For the stew:

- 1 can (14 oz) coconut milk
- 2 cups vegetable broth
- 2 large, sweet potatoes, cubed
- 1 can (15 oz) chickpeas
- 2 cups chopped kale or spinach
- 1 lb firm white fish (cod, halibut), cut into chunks
- Juice of 1 lime
- Fresh cilantro

METHOD

1. Heat olive oil in a large pot. Sauté onion until softened (5 minutes).
2. Add garlic, ginger, turmeric, cumin, and black pepper. Stir for 1 minute.
3. Add coconut milk, broth, and sweet potatoes. Bring to a boil.
4. Reduce heat and simmer for 15 minutes until sweet potatoes are tender.
5. Add chickpeas and kale. Simmer for 5 minutes.
6. Gently add fish chunks. Simmer for 5-7 minutes until fish is cooked through.
7. Remove from heat, add lime juice.
8. Serve in bowls, garnished with fresh cilantro.

THE SCIENCE Fish provides omega-3s that reduce cortisol surges (Frontiers in Psychology, 2020). Turmeric's curcumin lowers inflammatory cytokines (IL-6, TNF-alpha) elevated in PTSD. Sweet potatoes and greens provide magnesium that calms the nervous system. Coconut milk adds MCTs for brain support.

NUTRITIONAL HIGHLIGHTS ~340 calories per serving | Rich in: Omega-3s, Curcumin, Magnesium, Protein (22g)

VARIATIONS

- Vegetarian: Omit fish, double chickpeas
- Extra greens: Add more spinach or chard
- Spicier: Add cayenne pepper

STORAGE Refrigerate up to 4 days. Fish is best consumed within 2 days.

Freezes well without fish (add fresh when reheating).

7. ANXIETY-CALMING MAGNESIUM BOWL (Featured Recipe)

Nature's tranquilizer in whole-food form.

SERVES: 4 | **PREP:** 10 min | **COOK:** 25 min

WHY IT WORKS *This bowl is packed with magnesium—the mineral that regulates neurotransmitters and reduces cortisol. Perfect for anxiety, insomnia, and nervous tension. It combines pumpkin seeds, leafy greens, black beans, and avocado for maximum calming effect.*

INGREDIENTS

For the base:

- 1 cup quinoa
- 2 cups vegetable broth
- 1 can (15 oz) black beans, drained

For the bowl:

- 3 cups fresh spinach
- 1 avocado, sliced
- ¼ cup pumpkin seeds (pepitas)
- ¼ cup chopped almonds
- 1 cup cherry tomatoes, halved

For the dressing:

- 3 tablespoons tahini
- Juice of 1 lemon
- 2 tablespoons water
- 1 garlic clove, minced
- Salt and pepper

METHOD

1. Cook quinoa in vegetable broth according to package directions (about 15 minutes). Let cool slightly.
2. While quinoa cooks, toast pumpkin seeds, and almonds in a dry skil-let over medium heat until fragrant (3-4 minutes). Set aside.
3. In a small bowl, whisk together tahini, lemon juice, water, garlic, salt, and pepper. Add more water if needed to reach drizzling consistency.
4. Divide quinoa among four bowls.
5. Top each with black beans, fresh spinach, avocado slices, cherry tomatoes, toasted seeds, and almonds.
6. Drizzle with tahini dressing.

THE SCIENCE Magnesium calms the nervous system by regulating neurotransmitters and reducing cortisol (Nutrients, 2019). This bowl provides: pumpkin seeds (156mg magnesium per ¼ cup), spinach (157mg per cup cooked), black beans (60mg per ½ cup), almonds (80mg per ¼ cup). Total: ~450mg magnesium per serving (more than 100% daily value for women, 130% for men).

NUTRITIONAL HIGHLIGHTS ~480 calories per serving | Rich in: Magnesium (450mg), Fiber (15g), Protein (16g), Healthy fats

---

VARIATIONS

- Warm version: Sauté spinach until wilted
- Extra protein: Add grilled chicken or tofu
- Different greens: Use kale or Swiss chard (also high in magnesium)

STORAGE Components can be prepped ahead. Assemble fresh. Lasts 3 days refrigerated (keep avocado separate).

CLOSING: MEDICINE'S MISSING PIECE

When I work with patients, I see two kinds of medicine: the medicine that treats symptoms after disease arrives, and the medicine that prevents disease from arriving in the first place.

Pills can lower blood pressure—but food can prevent hypertension. Surgery can bypass clogged arteries—but food can keep them open. Therapy can process trauma—but food can calm the body's alarm system. Medication can stabilize mood—but food can provide the biochemistry for neurotransmitters to work.

Food is not alternative medicine. It is foundational medicine. The patients in this chapter prove it:

- Helena built a wall against cancer recurrence with cruciferous vegetables and flaxseed
- Samuel reversed heart disease with olive oil, beans, and movement
- Rosa breathed easier with COPD through antioxidants and omega-3s
- Elena lifted depression when food gave her medication something to work with
- Hannah calmed anxiety by stabilizing blood sugar and adding magnesium
- My own ADHD journey and Jamal's focus returned when nutrition partnered with medication
- Michael found stability in bipolar disorder through structured meals
- Sofia's nightmares faded when food lowered her body's trauma alarm
- Daniel's compulsions quieted when omega-3s and magnesium reduced anxiety
- Lila's autism symptoms eased when gut health improved
- Laura broke free from emotional eating by addressing the emotions themselves
- Ethan escaped sugar addiction through structured intervention
- Jasmine healed body image by reframing food as fuel, not punishment

These stories are not miracles. They are biology responding to nutrition.

As a psychiatrist and physician, I have learned one unshakable truth: medication without food is incomplete. Pills can ease symptoms, but without nutrition, healing stalls. Surgery can save lives, but without food, disease often returns.

The most powerful interventions happen when we integrate medicine:

- Psychiatry + Nutrition
- Cardiology + Mediterranean eating
- Oncology + anti-inflammatory diets
- Therapy + gut-brain support

This is not either/or. This is both/and.

If you are struggling with chronic illness, mental health challenges, or emotional eating patterns, know this:

You are not broken. You are biology responding to environment.

When you change the environment—when you change your plate, your pantry, your daily rhythm—biology changes too.

Arteries open. Neurons heal. Inflammation calms. Mood stabilizes. Cravings fade. Energy returns.

Food is medicine. And medicine is food. If these patients can heal, so can you.

The prescription is simple: beans and greens, olive oil and fish, whole grains and berries, water and movement, therapy and medication working together.

Take it daily. Watch your life transform.

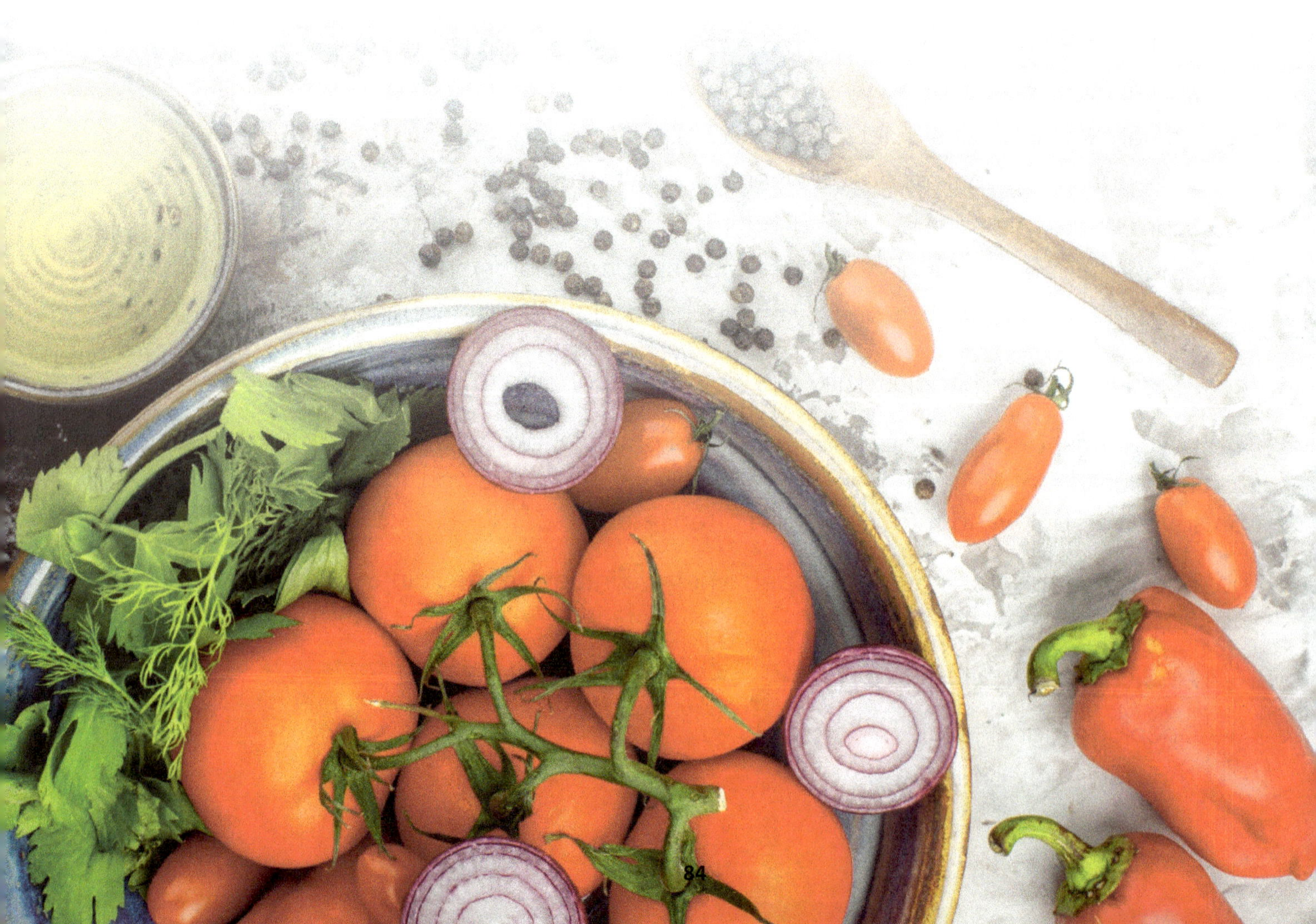

CHAPTER 4
The Science of Longevity

Reversing the Biological Clock

For centuries, aging was considered inevitable and unalterable. Today, science shows otherwise. While we cannot stop time, we can slow its effects and, in some cases, reverse biological aging markers.

Diet, combined with exercise, stress management, and modern interventions, creates the conditions for longer health spans—years lived in vitality, not just survival.

Aging research now focuses on three primary mechanisms:

- Telomere shortening — the erosion of chromosome caps that triggers cellular senescence
- Mitochondrial decline — the loss of energy powerhouses that accelerates fatigue and degeneration
- NAD+ depletion — the fall of a critical coenzyme that regulates DNA repair, metabolism, and longevity pathways

Alongside these are emerging therapies: peptides, hormones, stem cells, and precision nutrition. But the foundation remains unchanged: without nutrition, no peptide, stem cell therapy, or hormone can sustain lasting health.

This chapter explores the science of longevity, the evidence for reversal, and the practical strategies you can implement today—not decades from now.

PART A: THE THREE PILLARS OF LONGEVITY

Pillar 1: Telomeres — Protecting the Genetic Clock

Telomeres are the protective caps at the ends of chromosomes. With each cell division, telomeres shorten, eventually signaling cells to stop replicating. Shortened telomeres are strongly linked to cancer, cardiovascular disease, and accelerated aging.

Can We Lengthen Telomeres?

Yes. A landmark study in The Lancet Oncology (2008, Dean Ornish) showed that patients with early prostate cancer who adopted a plant-based diet, exercised, and managed stress increased their telomere length over five years.

This was the first evidence that telomeres could lengthen in humans.

Research from Harvard confirmed that diets rich in whole grains, nuts, legumes, and fruits are associated with longer telomeres, while processed meats and sugar shorten them.

What to Eat:

- Whole grains (oats, quinoa, barley)
- Nuts and seeds (walnuts, almonds, flaxseed)
- Legumes (beans, lentils, chickpeas)
- Fruits (especially berries)
- Leafy greens
- Omega-3-rich fish

What to Avoid:

- Processed meats
- Refined sugars
- Ultra-processed foods

CASE STUDY: Helena's Telomere Turnaround

Helena, fifty-five, was a corporate executive exhausted and fearful of her family history of early heart disease. Genetic testing showed her telomeres were shorter than average for her age—a marker of accelerated biological aging.

The Challenge: She felt like she was aging faster than her peers. She wanted to slow—or reverse—the process.

The Intervention: We rebuilt her lifestyle around telomere protection:

- Mediterranean diet: Beans, greens, olive oil, fish, nuts, whole grains
- Daily exercise: 30 minutes walking + strength training 3x/week
- Stress management: Meditation 10 minutes daily
- Sleep hygiene: 7-8 hours nightly
- Social connection: Joined a cooking club (Blue Zones principle)

The Results

- **Year 1:** Energy improved, cholesterol normalized

- **Year 2:** Telomere length stabilized (stopped shortening)
- **Year 3:** Follow-up testing showed slight telomere lengthening

Quote: "I feel like I bought back a decade. My body responded when I gave it what it needed."

The Science: Helena's recovery reflects the Ornish study: while genetics matter, lifestyle—especially diet—decides how fast the clock ticks.

The Lesson: Telomeres are not fixed. With consistent nutrition and lifestyle, biological aging can be slowed and even partially reversed.

Pillar 2: Mitochondria — Energizing Longevity

Mitochondria are tiny powerhouses inside cells, producing ATP, the energy currency of life. When mitochondria falter, we see fatigue, muscle loss, cognitive decline, and diseases like Parkinson's and Alzheimer's.

Can We Restore Mitochondrial Function?

Yes. Through nutrition and lifestyle interventions. Nutritional Mitochondrial Support:

- Polyphenols: Found in berries, green tea, and red wine (resveratrol), they protect mitochondria from oxidative stress
- Coenzyme Q10 (CoQ10): Found in fish, nuts, and whole grains, it supports the electron transport chain
- Alpha-lipoic acid: Present in spinach and broccoli, it helps regenerate antioxidants
- Omega-3s: Improve mitochondrial membrane fluidity and efficiency
- PQQ (Pyrroloquinoline quinone): Found in fermented foods, promotes mitochondrial biogenesis (creation of new mitochondria)

CASE STUDY: Tomas and Chronic Fatigue Reversal

Tomas, forty-eight, was an engineer diagnosed with chronic fatigue. He lived on processed foods and rarely ate vegetables. Despite adequate sleep, he felt exhausted constantly.

The Challenge: His fatigue was so severe he could barely climb stairs without breathlessness. Standard medical workup showed no deficiencies.

The Intervention: We introduced a mitochondrial-supportive diet:

- Blueberries daily: (polyphenols protect mitochondria)
- Salmon 3x/week: (omega-3s improve mitochondrial function)
- Green tea: (EGCG supports energy production)

- Walnuts and spinach: (alpha-lipoic acid, vitamin E)
- CoQ10 supplementation: 100mg daily (with cardiologist approval)

Exercise: Started with 10-minute walks, gradually increased

The Results

- **Month 3:** Energy noticeably improved
- **Month 6:** Fatigue dramatically reduced, could climb stairs without breathlessness
- **Year 1:** Returned to weekend hiking

Quote: "I didn't realize how much my diet was draining me. Now I feel alive again."

The Science: Tomas' transformation reflected research from Aging Cell journal: mitochondrial health can be preserved—and partially restored—through diet and exercise.

The Lesson: Fatigue is not always a disease to diagnose—sometimes it is biology starving for the right nutrients.

Pillar 3: NAD+ — The Master Regulator of Aging

Nicotinamide adenine dinucleotide (NAD+) is a coenzyme found in all living cells. It regulates:

- DNA repair
- Energy metabolism
- Sirtuin activity (proteins tied to longevity)

NAD+ declines with age, and low NAD+ is associated with metabolic dys-function, neurodegeneration, and cancer risk.

Can We Boost NAD+?

Yes, through diet, fasting, exercise, and supplementation.

Boosting NAD+ Naturally:

- Caloric restriction and intermittent fasting: Increase NAD+ availability
- Nicotinamide riboside (NR) and nicotinamide mononucleotide (NMN): NAD+ precursors under intense study
- Foods rich in tryptophan and niacin: Turkey, peanuts, mushrooms, avocados
- Polyphenols in grapes and pomegranates: Activate sirtuins, enhancing NAD+ pathways

Exercise: Increases NAD+ production naturally

Research Highlights:

- Cell Metabolism (2016): Supplementation with NMN improved mitochondrial function and glucose tolerance in mice
- Nature Communications (2019): NAD+ precursors improved muscle function in elderly volunteers

CASE STUDY: Alan's Midlife Renewal

Alan, fifty-two, felt "older than his years." He was prediabetic, overweight, and constantly fatigued. He described himself as "running on empty."

The Challenge: Standard interventions (diet advice, exercise recommendations) had failed. He needed a more targeted approach.

The Intervention: We emphasized NAD+-supportive strategies: Diet rich in NAD+ precursors:

- Turkey and chicken (tryptophan)
- Peanuts and peanut butter (niacin)
- Mushrooms (niacin, B-vitamins)
- Pomegranates (polyphenols activate sirtuins)

Intermittent fasting: 16:8 pattern (16 hours fasting, 8-hour eating window) 3 days/week

NMN supplementation: 250mg daily (with physician guidance) Exercise: Strength training 3x/week (increases NAD+ naturally)

The Results

- **Month 6:** Lost 15 pounds, energy improved
- **Year 1:** Lost 20 pounds, glucose normalized, energy "like I am 40 again"

Lab work: Improved insulin sensitivity, lower inflammatory markers

Quote: "I feel like I turned back the clock. My body finally has the fuel it needs."

The Science: Alan's recovery reflects emerging NAD+ research: restoration can delay age-related metabolic decline and improve energy production.

The Lesson: NAD+ is the cellular currency of youth. When we restore it through diet, fasting, and targeted supplementation, the body regenerates.

PART B: REGENERATIVE TOOLS & PRECISION NUTRITION

Stem Cells and Nutrition: Regeneration from Within

Stem cells can differentiate into many types of tissues, offering potential to repair joints, regenerate skin, and restore organs. With age, stem cells decline in number and function. Nutrition directly influences their vitality.

How Nutrition Supports Stem Cells:

- Polyphenols (berries, olive oil, green tea) activate pathways that extend stem cell function
- Vitamin D is essential for stem cell differentiation into bone, muscle, and immune cells
- Omega-3 fatty acids reduce inflammation, allowing stem cells to regenerate tissue
- Fasting and caloric restriction increase circulating stem cells and enhance regeneration

Research Evidence:

- Cell Stem Cell (2014, Longo et al.): Fasting cycles promoted stem cell-based regeneration of the immune system
- Stem Cell Reports (2018): Omega-3s improved mesenchymal stem cell differentiation and proliferation

CASE STUDY: Julian's Knee Recovery

Julian, sixty-one, was a former runner suffering from severe knee osteoarthritis. He underwent stem cell therapy but wanted to maximize results.

The Challenge: Stem cell therapy alone has variable success. Nutrition could enhance the healing environment.

The Intervention: Julian adopted an anti-inflammatory, stem-cell-supportive diet:

- Salmon 4x/week: (omega-3s reduce inflammation)
- Olive oil as primary fat: (polyphenols support stem cell function)
- Turmeric daily: (curcumin reduces joint inflammation)
- Leafy greens: (vitamin K, magnesium for bone health)

The Results

- **Month 3:** Swelling reduced, mobility improved
- **Month 6:** Recovery faster than physician expected Year 1: Returned to hiking

Quote: "My doctor said my stem cells 'took better than most.' I believe the diet made the difference."

The Science: Julian's outcome highlights the constructive collaboration between regenerative medicine and nutrition. Stem cells need the right environment to thrive—and food creates that environment.

The Lesson: Regenerative therapies work best when the body is nutritionally prepared to support healing.

Peptides: Targeted Healing Molecules

Peptides—short chains of amino acids—regulate many biological functions. Emerging peptide therapies aim to accelerate healing, reduce inflammation, and even extend lifespan.

Promising Peptides:

- BPC-157: Promotes tissue repair, reduces inflammation (especially tendons, gut lining)
- Thymosin Alpha-1: Enhances immune function
- Epitalon: Linked to telomere extension in animal studies
- GHK-Cu: Improves skin regeneration and hair growth

Research Highlights:

- Peptides (2018): BPC-157 accelerated tendon healing in animal models
- Rejuvenation Research (2019): Epitalon extended lifespan in rodents
- Journal of Immunology (2017): Thymosin Alpha-1 improved immune resilience in viral infections

CASE STUDY: Karen's Shoulder Recovery

Karen, forty-five, was a professional violinist who developed a severe shoulder injury. Physical therapy had failed.

The Challenge: Without recovery, her career was over.

The Intervention: Karen's physician prescribed BPC-157 (via injection) alongside:

Anti-inflammatory nutrition:

- Salmon and sardines (omega-3s)
- Turmeric and ginger (curcumin, gingerol)
- Leafy greens (magnesium)
- Bone broth (collagen, amino acids)

Physical therapy: Gradual range-of-motion exercises

The Results

- **Month 2:** Pain significantly reduced
- **Month 3:** Range of motion restored Month 6: Returned to performing

Quote: "The peptide helped, but I believe the nutrition created the environment for healing."

The Science: Karen's case reflects how peptides bridge the gap between nutrition and regenerative medicine. BPC-157 accelerated tissue repair, while nutrition provided the building blocks.

The Lesson: Peptides are powerful tools—but they work best when paired with foundational nutrition.

Fasting: The Ancient Regenerative Tool

Fasting is one of the oldest practices in human history, now confirmed by modern science as a regenerative tool.

Mechanisms of Fasting:

- Autophagy: The cellular "cleanup" process, triggered by fasting, recycles damaged proteins
- Stem cell activation: Prolonged fasting regenerates immune cells
- Insulin sensitivity: Fasting improves glucose metabolism
- Inflammation reduction: Fasting lowers inflammatory markers

Research Evidence:

- Science Translational Medicine (2015, Longo et al.): Fasting cycles rejuvenated the immune system in mice and humans
- Cell Metabolism (2019): Intermittent fasting reduced cardiovascular risk factors and improved cognition
- New England Journal of Medicine (2019): Fasting reduced inflammation, blood pressure, and oxidative stress

Types of Fasting:

- Intermittent fasting (IF): 16:8 (16 hours fasting, 8-hour eating window) or 5:2 (5 days normal eating, 2 days reduced calories)
- Prolonged fasting: 2-4 days (under medical supervision)
- Fasting-mimicking diet (FMD): Developed by Valter Longo, replicates fasting effects while allowing lesser amounts of plant-based calories

CASE STUDY: Ethan's Immune Reset

Ethan, fifty-two, struggled with recurrent infections and fatigue. Despite adequate sleep and decent diet, he felt constantly worn down.

The Challenge: His immune system seemed weakened, but standard tests showed no deficiencies.

The Intervention: With medical supervision, Ethan adopted a fasting-mimicking diet for 5 days each month:

Days 1-5:

- 800-1,100 calories daily
- Plant-based: vegetable soups, nuts, olive oil, herbal teas
- No animal products, minimal protein

Days 6-30:

- Mediterranean diet: beans, greens, fish, olive oil, whole grains

The Results

- **Month 3:** Infections decreased
- **Month 6:** Blood markers of inflammation (CRP, IL-6) decreased
- **Year 1:** Energy significantly improved, no infections for 9 months

Quote: "I didn't believe fasting could 'reset' my immune system, but the results speak for themselves."

The Science: Ethan's improvement echoes published research: fasting strengthens immunity and promotes cellular regeneration (Science Translational Medicine, 2015).

The Lesson: Fasting is not starvation—it is strategic cellular renewal. When done safely, it activates the body's innate healing systems.

Precision Nutrition: The Future Is Personal

Precision nutrition goes beyond "eat more vegetables." It personalizes food choices based on genetics, microbiome composition, and metabolic responses.

Tools of Precision Nutrition:

- Continuous glucose monitors (CGMs): Reveal how individual bodies respond to specific foods
- Microbiome testing: Names gut bacteria composition and personalized food recommendations
- Genetic testing: Reveals predispositions (e.g., caffeine metabolism, lactose intolerance, omega-3 conversion efficiency)

- Biomarker panels: Track inflammation, hormones, nutrient status

Research Evidence:

- Cell (2015, Zeevi et al.): Two people can have opposite blood sugar responses to the same food. Personalized diets based on gut microbiota predicted better outcomes than standard guidelines.
- Nature Medicine (2019): Precision nutrition interventions improved glycemic control in prediabetic patients by tailoring meals to their responses.

CASE STUDY: Jordan's Data-Driven Diet

Jordan, thirty-five, was an entrepreneur struggling with fatigue despite "eating healthy."

The Challenge: He followed general nutrition advice but still felt exhausted, brain-fogged, and struggled with weight.

The Intervention: Jordan used precision nutrition tools:

- Continuous glucose monitor (CGM): Revealed that oatmeal (healthy) spiked his glucose, while sweet potatoes did not
- Microbiome test: Showed low diversity and overabundance of inflammation-promoting bacteria

Personalized adjustments:

- Replaced oatmeal with lentils for breakfast
- Added fermented foods daily (kefir, sauerkraut)
- Increased fiber from vegetables and beans
- Reduced foods that spiked his glucose

The Results

- **Month 3:** Energy stabilized, brain fog lifted
- **Month 6:** Lost 10 pounds without calorie counting

Quote: "I thought I was eating healthy. Turns out, my body needed something different. Data showed me the way."

The Science: Jordan's story reflects the power of precision nutrition: no two bodies respond the same way. Personalization improves results.

The Lesson: General nutrition advice is a starting point. Precision tools reveal what YOUR body needs.

The Gut Microbiome: The Hidden Organ of Longevity

The gut microbiome—trillions of bacteria in the digestive tract—influences immunity, mood, metabolism, and longevity.

How Microbiome Affects Longevity:

- Diversity = Health: Greater bacterial diversity correlates with longer lifespan (Nature, 2016)
- Centenarians have unique microbes: That produce anti-inflammatory compounds (Cell Host & Microbe, 2020)
- Microbiome transplants: Improve insulin sensitivity in metabolic syndrome patients (Science, 2018)

Foods That Feed the Microbiome:

- Prebiotics: Fibers in garlic, onions, asparagus, bananas
- Probiotics: Kefir, yogurt, sauerkraut, kimchi, miso
- Polyphenols: Berries, green tea, dark chocolate, olive oil

CASE STUDY: Amelia's Microbiome Makeover

Amelia, forty-eight, struggled with IBS and depression. She had low micro-biome diversity (confirmed by testing).

The Challenge: Her gut issues worsened her mood, and her mood worsened her gut issues—a vicious cycle.

The Intervention: We focused on rebuilding microbiome diversity:

- Fermented foods daily: Kefir, sauerkraut, kimchi (probiotics)
- High-fiber diet: Beans, lentils, vegetables, whole grains (prebiotics)
- Polyphenol-rich foods: Berries, green tea, dark chocolate (feed beneficial bacteria)

Eliminated: Ultra-processed foods (damage microbiome)

The Results

- **Month 3:** IBS flares decreased significantly
- **Month 6:** Mood improved, anxiety reduced

Microbiome retest: Diversity increased by 40%

Quote: "Fixing my gut fixed my mind. I didn't realize how connected they were."

The Science: Amelia's recovery reflects Psychiatry Research (2019): probiotics reduced anxiety symptoms by 20-30% by improving gut-brain communication.

The Lesson: The gut is the second brain. When we nourish it, mental and physical health follow.

PART C: Blue Zones & LONGEVITY WISDOM

What Centenarians Teach Us

The five Blue Zones—Okinawa, Sardinia, Ikaria, Nicoya, and Loma Linda—offer living laboratories for longevity. People in these regions live 7-10 years longer on average and have 70-80% lower chronic disease rates.

Shared Principles:

1. Plant-based diets: 90-95% of calories from plants
2. Beans daily: Lentils, chickpeas, soy, black beans
3. Healthy fats: Olive oil, nuts, seeds
4. Low sugar, minimal processed foods
5. Natural movement: Walking, gardening integrated into daily life
6. Community connection: Eating with others, strong social ties
7. Purpose (Ikigai in Okinawa): Reason to wake up each morning

Research Evidence:

- Journal of Aging Research (2016): Centenarians in Ikaria had lower inflammation markers and better cardiovascular profiles than age-matched peers elsewhere
- American Journal of Clinical Nutrition (2018): Blue Zones dietary patterns associated with 30-50% reduction in all-cause mortality

Biohacking Blue Zones Wisdom

Today, we can "biohack" Blue Zones wisdom by combining traditional practices with modern science.

Modern Applications:

- Use wearables: Track activity, sleep, and glucose responses
- Add supplements: Omega-3s, curcumin, NAD+ precursors (to enhance whole-food diets)
- Practice structured fasting: To mimic Blue Zones calorie patterns (they eat less overall)
- Track biomarkers: To measure progress objectively
- Join communities: Cooking clubs, walking groups (replicates Blue Zones social connection)

SECTION 3: THE 30-DAY LONGEVITY PLAN

GOAL: Slow biological aging, enhance vitality, extend health span

FOCUS: Telomere protection, mitochondrial support, NAD+ boosting, gut health, anti-inflammatory eating

WEEK 1: RESET THE BODY

Daily Structure:

- Eliminate: Processed foods, refined sugars, excessive alcohol
- Emphasize: Beans, vegetables, whole grains, olive oil, water
- Add: Omega-3s (fish or flax), Vitamin D supplementation

Sample Days:

Day 1:

- Breakfast: Oatmeal + blueberries + walnuts
- Lunch: Lentil soup + whole grain bread
- Dinner: Salmon + spinach + quinoa
- Practice: 30-minute walk, 8 glasses water

Day 2:

- Breakfast: Greek yogurt + raspberries + almonds
- Lunch: Chickpea salad + olive oil
- Dinner: Cod + kale + sweet potato
- Practice: Strength training (20 min), begin food journal

Continue pattern through Day 7

WEEK 2: MITOCHONDRIAL BOOST

Daily Structure:

- Add: Daily polyphenols (blueberries, green tea, pomegranate)
- Include: CoQ10-rich foods (fish, nuts, whole grains)
- Begin: 14-hour overnight fast (finish dinner by 7 PM, breakfast at 9 AM)
- Exercise: Strength training 2x, aerobic 3x

Sample Days:

Day 8:

- Breakfast: Chia pudding + pomegranate
- Lunch: Sardinian minestrone
- Dinner: Grilled salmon + roasted vegetables

- Practice: 16-hour fast (experimental), green tea 2x

Day 9:

- Breakfast: Smoothie (kefir + berries + spinach)
- Lunch: Mediterranean grain bowl
- Dinner: Turmeric lentils + arugula
- Practice: Strength training, meditation 10 min

Continue pattern through Day 14

WEEK 3: STEM CELL ACTIVATION & NAD+ BOOST

Daily Structure:

- Introduce: Fasting-mimicking protocol 3-5 days (under medical guidance)
    - 800-1,100 calories/day
    - Plant-based: vegetable soups, nuts, herbal teas
- Emphasize: NAD+-supporting foods (mushrooms, turkey, peanuts, pomegranates)
- Add: NMN or NR supplementation (with physician guidance)
- Practice: Deep sleep hygiene (7-8 hours nightly)

***Fasting-Mimicking (Days 15–17 or 15–19):* Each day:**

- Breakfast: Herbal tea + small handful nuts
- Lunch: Vegetable soup (tomato, celery, carrots, olive oil)
- Dinner: Steamed vegetables + avocado + olive oil
- Snack: Olives, herbal tea

Non-Fasting Days (18-21 or 20-21):

- Return to Week 1-2 pattern
- Emphasize nutrient density to replenish

WEEK 4: LONGEVITY LIFESTYLE

Daily Structure:

- Maintain: Plant-based majority diet (90% plants, 10% animal if desired)
- Continue: Fermented foods daily (kefir, sauerkraut, miso)
- Allow: Dark chocolate (70%+) and red wine in moderation
- Practice: 14-16-hour overnight fasts most days
- Exercise: Balanced training (aerobic, strength, flexibility)
- Social: Share meals with others 3x this week

Sample Days:

Day 22:

- Breakfast: Oatmeal + flaxseed + berries
- Lunch: Black bean bowl + avocado
- Dinner: Sardines + roasted vegetables
- Practice: Pilates class, cook with family

Day 28:

- Breakfast: Smoothie (kefir + greens + chia)
- Lunch: Mediterranean grain bowl
- Dinner: Salmon + Brussels sprouts + quinoa
- Practice: Gratitude journaling, early bedtime

Day 30: REFLECTION

- Measure progress: Energy, sleep, mood, weight, lab markers if available
- Write personal longevity vision
- Commit to 3 habits to support long-term

SECTION 4: SEVEN LONGEVITY RECIPES

1. TELOMERE-PROTECTING SALAD (Featured Recipe)

Whole foods that lengthen your genetic clock.

SERVES: 4 | **PREP:** 15 min | **COOK:** 0 min

WHY IT WORKS: *This salad combines foods scientifically linked to longer telomeres: leafy greens, berries, walnuts, and olive oil. Perfect for cellular antiaging.*

INGREDIENTS

For the base:

- 4 cups mixed greens (kale, spinach, arugula)
- 2 cups baby spinach
- 1 cup fresh blueberries
- ½ cup chopped walnuts
- ¼ cup pomegranate seeds

For the dressing:

- 3 tablespoons extra virgin olive oil
- 1 tablespoon balsamic vinegar
- 1 teaspoon Dijon mustard
- 1 garlic clove, minced
- Salt and pepper

METHOD

1. In a large bowl, combine all greens.
2. Add blueberries, walnuts, and pomegranate seeds.
3. In a small bowl, whisk together olive oil, vinegar, mustard, garlic, salt, and pepper.
4. Pour dressing over salad and toss gently.
5. Serve at once.

THE SCIENCE: The Lancet Oncology (2008): Plant-based diets increased telomere length in prostate cancer patients. Blueberries provide anthocyanins that protect DNA. Walnuts supply omega-3s linked to longer telomeres (American Journal of Clinical Nutrition, 2021). Olive oil polyphenols reduce oxidative stress.

NUTRITIONAL HIGHLIGHTS: ~220 calories per serving | Rich in: Antioxidants, Omega-3s, Fiber (6g), Polyphenols

VARIATIONS

- Extra protein: Add grilled chicken or chickpeas
- Different berries: Use strawberries or raspberries
- Seed boost: Add chia or hemp seeds

STORAGE: Best fresh. Keep dressing separate if meal-prepping components.

2. MITOCHONDRIAL GREEN SMOOTHIE (Featured Recipe)

Power up your cellular engines.

SERVES: 2 | **PREP:** 5 min | **COOK:** 0 min

WHY IT WORKS: *This smoothie delivers nutrients that specifically support mitochondrial function: polyphenols from berries, omega-3 precursors from chia, and antioxidants from spinach.*

INGREDIENTS

- 2 cups fresh spinach
- 1 cup frozen blueberries
- 1 banana
- 2 tablespoons chia seeds
- 1 tablespoon ground flaxseed
- 1 cup unsweetened almond milk
- ½ cup cooled green tea (optional: for extra polyphenols)
- Ice cubes

METHOD

1. Add all ingredients to blender.
2. Blend on high until completely smooth (1-2 minutes).
3. Add ice and blend again if desired thickness.
4. Pour into glasses and serve at once.

THE SCIENCE: Aging Cell (2014): Polyphenols and omega-3s preserved mitochondrial efficiency. Blueberries provide pterostilbene and anthocya-nins that protect mitochondria. Chia and flax provide alpha-linolenic acid (plant omega-3). Green tea's EGCG enhances cellular energy production.

NUTRITIONAL HIGHLIGHTS: ~240 calories per serving | Rich in: Polyphenols, Omega-3 precursors, Fiber (10g), Antioxidants

---

VARIATIONS

- Extra protein: Add protein powder or Greek yogurt
- Different greens: Use kale or Swiss chard
- Creamier: Add avocado

STORAGE: Best fresh. Can refrigerate up to 24 hours (shake before drinking).

3. NAD+-SUPPORTING MUSHROOM BOWL (Featured Recipe)

Fuel your longevity pathways with niacin-rich foods.

SERVES: 4 | **PREP:** 10 min | **COOK:** 25 min

WHY IT WORKS: *This bowl is designed to boost NAD+ through ni-acin-rich mushrooms, tryptophan from chickpeas, and sirtuin-activating polyphenols from olive oil. Perfect for cellular repair and energy.*

INGREDIENTS

For the base:

- 1 cup quinoa
- 2 cups vegetable broth

For the bowl:

- 3 cups mixed mushrooms (cremini, shiitake, portobello), sliced
- 1 can (15 oz) chickpeas, drained
- 2 cups fresh spinach
- ¼ cup chopped walnuts
- 2 tablespoons fresh parsley

For cooking:

- 3 tablespoons extra virgin olive oil
- 3 garlic cloves, minced
- 1 teaspoon dried thyme
- Salt and pepper
- Juice of 1 lemon

METHOD

1. Cook quinoa in vegetable broth according to package directions (about 15 minutes).
2. While quinoa cooks, heat 2 tablespoons olive oil in a large skillet over medium-high heat.
3. Add mushrooms and cook until browned and tender (7-8 minutes). Season with salt, pepper, and thyme.
4. Add garlic and cook for 1 minute.
5. Add chickpeas and spinach. Cook until spinach wilts (2 minutes).
6. Divide quinoa among four bowls.
7. Top with mushroom-chickpea mixture, walnuts, and fresh parsley.
8. Drizzle with remaining olive oil and lemon juice.

THE SCIENCE: Mushrooms are rich in niacin (vitamin B3), a direct NAD+ precursor. Chickpeas provide tryptophan (converted to NAD+). Olive oil polyphenols activate sirtuins, which depend on NAD+ for longevity effects (Cell Metabolism, 2016). Quinoa provides complete protein for cellular repair.

NUTRITIONAL HIGHLIGHTS: ~380 calories per serving | Rich in: Niacin (6mg), Protein (14g), Fiber (10g), Polyphenols

VARIATIONS

- Extra NAD+ boost: Add turkey or chicken (high in tryptophan)
- Different grain: Use brown rice or barley
- Vegan: Perfect as is

STORAGE: Refrigerate up to 4 days. Reheat gently or serve at room temperature.

4. STEM CELL REGENERATION STEW (Featured Recipe)

Create the environment for cellular renewal.

SERVES: 6 | **PREP:** 15 min | **COOK:** 40 min

WHY IT WORKS: *This stew combines omega-3s, vitamin D, and anti-in-flammatory compounds that support stem cell function and tissue regeneration. Perfect for recovery and longevity.*

INGREDIENTS

For the base:

- 2 tablespoons olive oil
- 1 onion, diced
- 3 garlic cloves, minced
- 1 tablespoon fresh ginger, grated

For the stew:

- 2 large, sweet potatoes, cubed
- 2 carrots, sliced
- 1 can (15 oz) white beans
- 1 can (14 oz) diced tomatoes
- 4 cups vegetable broth
- 1 can (14 oz) coconut milk
- 2 cups chopped kale
- 1 lb firm white fish (cod, halibut), cut into chunks
- 1 teaspoon turmeric
- 1 teaspoon cumin
- ½ teaspoon black pepper
- Salt to taste

To finish:

- Juice of 1 lime
- Fresh cilantro

METHOD

1. Heat olive oil in a large pot. Sauté onion until softened (5 minutes).
2. Add garlic, ginger, turmeric, cumin, and black pepper. Stir for 1 minute.
3. Add sweet potatoes, carrots, beans, tomatoes, and broth. Bring to a boil.
4. Reduce heat and simmer for 20 minutes until vegetables are tender.
5. Add coconut milk and kale. Simmer for 5 minutes.
6. Gently add fish chunks. Simmer for 5-7 minutes until fish is cooked through.
7. Remove from heat, add lime juice.
8. Serve garnished with fresh cilantro.

THE SCIENCE: Fish provides omega-3s that improve stem cell differentiation (Stem Cell Reports, 2018). Vitamin D (from fish) is essential for stem cell function. Sweet potatoes and carrots provide beta-carotene (vitamin A precursor) necessary for tissue regeneration. Turmeric's curcumin reduces inflammation that impairs stem cell activity.

NUTRITIONAL HIGHLIGHTS: ~350 calories per serving | Rich in: Omega-3s, Vitamin D, Vitamin A, Protein (24g)

VARIATIONS

- Vegetarian: Omit fish, double beans, add tofu
- Extra anti-inflammatory: Add more turmeric and ginger
- Different greens: Use spinach or Swiss chard

STORAGE: Refrigerate up to 4 days (fish best within 2 days). Freezes well without fish.

5. Blue Zones LONGEVITY BOWL (Featured Recipe)

Eat like a centenarian.

SERVES: 4 | **PREP:** 10 min (if components pre-cooked) | **COOK:** 0 min

WHY IT WORKS: *This bowl replicates the dietary patterns of Okinawa, Sardinia, and Ikaria: beans, whole grains, vegetables, nuts, and olive oil. The exact combination associated with living past 100.*

INGREDIENTS

For the base:

- 2 cups cooked barley or brown rice
- 1 can (15 oz) black beans or chickpeas, drained

For the bowl:

- 2 cups mixed greens (spinach, arugula, kale)
- 1 cup cherry tomatoes, halved
- 1 cucumber, diced
- ½ red onion, thinly sliced
- ¼ cup Kalamata olives
- ¼ cup chopped walnuts
- 2 tablespoons pumpkin seeds

For the dressing:

- 3 tablespoons extra virgin olive oil
- Juice of 1 lemon
- 1 teaspoon dried oregano
- 1 garlic clove, minced
- Salt and pepper

METHOD

1. Divide barley or rice among four bowls.
2. Top each with beans, mixed greens, tomatoes, cucumber, onion, and olives.
3. Sprinkle with walnuts and pumpkin seeds.
4. In a small bowl, whisk together olive oil, lemon juice, oregano, garlic, salt, and pepper.
5. Drizzle dressing over each bowl.
6. Serve at room temperature or chilled.

THE SCIENCE: This bowl mirrors Blue Zones eating patterns associated with 7-10 years longer lifespan (Journal of Aging Research, 2016). Beans provide resistant starch and protein. Whole grains lower cholesterol. Leafy greens provide folate and nitrates for vascular health. Walnuts and olive oil provide healthy fats. The combination reduces inflammation and oxidative stress.

NUTRITIONAL HIGHLIGHTS: ~420 calories per serving | Rich in: Fiber (14g), Protein (13g), Healthy fats, Antioxidants

VARIATIONS

- Warm version: Heat grains and beans before assembling
- Extra protein: Add grilled fish or tofu
- Seasonal: Add roasted vegetables in winter

STORAGE: Components can be prepped ahead. Dress just before serving. Lasts 4 days refrigerated.

6. FASTING-RECOVERY BONE BROTH (Featured Recipe)

Nourish and rebuild after fasting periods.

SERVES: 6-8 | **PREP:** 15 min | **COOK:** 4-24 hours

WHY IT WORKS: *Bone broth provides collagen, amino acids, and minerals that support tissue repair and gut healing—perfect for breaking fasts or supporting regeneration. Rich in glycine and proline for cellular repair.*

INGREDIENTS

For the broth:

- 2-3 lbs bones (chicken, beef, or fish bones)
- 2 tablespoons apple cider vinegar (helps extract minerals)
- 1 onion, quartered
- 3 carrots, chopped
- 3 celery stalks, chopped
- 4 garlic cloves, smashed
- 2 bay leaves
- 1 tablespoon peppercorns
- Fresh herbs (parsley, thyme, rosemary)
- 12-16 cups water

To finish:

- Salt to taste
- Fresh lemon juice
- Optional: turmeric, ginger for anti-inflammatory boost

METHOD

Stovetop Method (12-24 hours):

1. Place bones in a large pot. Add vinegar and let sit for 30 minutes (extracts minerals).
2. Add vegetables, herbs, peppercorns, and water. Bring to a boil.
3. Reduce heat to lowest simmer. Cook for 12-24 hours, skimming foam occasionally.
4. Strain through fine-mesh sieve.
5. Season with salt and lemon juice.

Instant Pot Method (3-4 hours):

1. Place all ingredients in Instant Pot.
2. Cook on high pressure for 3-4 hours.
3. Natural release, then strain.

Slow Cooker Method (12-24 hours):

1. Place all ingredients in slow cooker.
2. Cook on low for 12-24 hours.
3. Strain and season.

THE SCIENCE: Bone broth provides collagen (breaks down into gelatin), glycine and proline (amino acids for tissue repair), and minerals (calcium, magnesium, phosphorus). Glycine supports gut lining repair and has anti-inflammatory effects (Nutrients, 2019). Perfect for post-fasting cellular rebuilding.

NUTRITIONAL HIGHLIGHTS: ~40 calories per cup | Rich in: Collagen peptides, Glycine, Minerals

VARIATIONS

- Add turmeric and ginger: Boosts anti-inflammatory properties
- Vegetable version: Use mushroom stems, seaweed, miso for vegan alternative
- Healing additions: Add fresh garlic and ginger when reheating

STORAGE: Refrigerate up to 5 days (fat will solidify on top—remove or leave for cooking fat). Freezes beautifully for 6 months in portions.

7. RESVERATROL-RICH BERRY COMPOTE (Featured Recipe)

Activate your longevity genes with every spoonful.

SERVES: 8 | **PREP:** 5 min | **COOK:** 20 min

WHY IT WORKS: *This compote concentrates polyphenols from berries—particularly resveratrol and anthocyanins—that activate sirtuins (longevity genes) and protect against cellular aging. Perfect over yogurt, oatmeal, or as a dessert.*

INGREDIENTS

- 2 cups fresh or frozen blueberries
- 2 cups fresh or frozen strawberries, sliced
- 1 cup fresh or frozen raspberries
- 1 cup fresh or frozen blackberries
- ¼ cup water
- 2 tablespoons lemon juice
- 1 tablespoon chia seeds
- Optional: 1-2 tablespoons honey or maple syrup (if berries are tart)
- Pinch of cinnamon

METHOD

1. In a medium saucepan, combine all berries and water.
2. Bring to a simmer over medium heat.
3. Cook for 15-20 minutes, stirring occasionally, until berries break down and mixture thickens.
4. Mash berries lightly with a potato masher or fork (leave some chunks for texture).
5. Stir in chia seeds, lemon juice, and cinnamon.
6. Remove from heat and let cool (chia will thicken the compote further).
7. Taste and add sweetener if desired.

THE SCIENCE: Berries are among the richest sources of polyphenols, particularly anthocyanins and resveratrol, which activate sirtuins—proteins that regulate cellular aging (Cell, 2013). Blueberries improve memory and protect neurons (Nutrients, 2020). Strawberries and raspberries reduce oxidative stress and inflammation. Chia adds omega-3s and fiber.

NUTRITIONAL HIGHLIGHTS: ~70 calories per ¼ cup | Rich in: An-thocyanins, Resveratrol, Vitamin C, Fiber (4g)

VARIATIONS

- Serve over: Greek yogurt, overnight oats, chia pudding
- Dessert version: Top with dark chocolate shavings
- Savory application: Use as glaze for salmon or chicken

STORAGE: Refrigerate up to 2 weeks. Freezes well for 6 months.

CLOSING: THE FUTURE YOU CAN LIVE TODAY

The future of longevity is not science fiction. It is unfolding in labs, clinics, and kitchens worldwide.

Fasting regenerates cells. Precision nutrition tailors food to the individual. NAD+ boosters and peptides extend vitality. Stem cells and gene editing push the frontier of what is possible.

But the future is not only about advanced technology. It is about merging ancient wisdom with innovative science.

The Blue Zones show us that longevity comes from:

- Beans eaten daily
- Movement woven into life
- Community at the table
- Purpose each morning

When we combine this wisdom with:

- Intermittent fasting
- Microbiome testing
- NAD+ optimization
- Anti-inflammatory nutrition

...we create a complete longevity strategy.

The patients in this chapter prove it works:

- Helena lengthened her telomeres through diet and lifestyle
- Tomas restored mitochondrial function and reclaimed energy
- Alan boosted NAD+ and reversed prediabetes
- Julian's stem cells thrived in an anti-inflammatory environment
- Karen healed her shoulder with peptides plus nutrition
- Ethan reset his immune system through fasting
- Jordan discovered his unique metabolic needs through precision tools
- Amelia rebuilt her microbiome and lifted depression

These are not outliers. They are biology responding to the right inputs.

If I could overcome ADHD, exhaustion, and family history with food and movement...

If my husband reversed hypertension in three months...

If patients can lengthen telomeres, restore mitochondria, and regenerate stem cells...

Then so can you.

The choice to regenerate begins not in a lab, but on your plate.

You do not need to wait for gene therapy or future breakthroughs. The tools are here:

- Beans and greens
- Olive oil and berries
- Fasting and movement
- Community and purpose
- Sleep and stress management

From there, the future opens.

Telomeres lengthen. Mitochondria energize. NAD+ restores. Stem cells regenerate. The biological clock slows—and in some measures, reverses.

This is not theory. This is evidence.

This is your potential.

The science is clear. The stories are real. The choice is yours.

Choose regeneration. Choose vitality. Choose to live not just longer, but better.

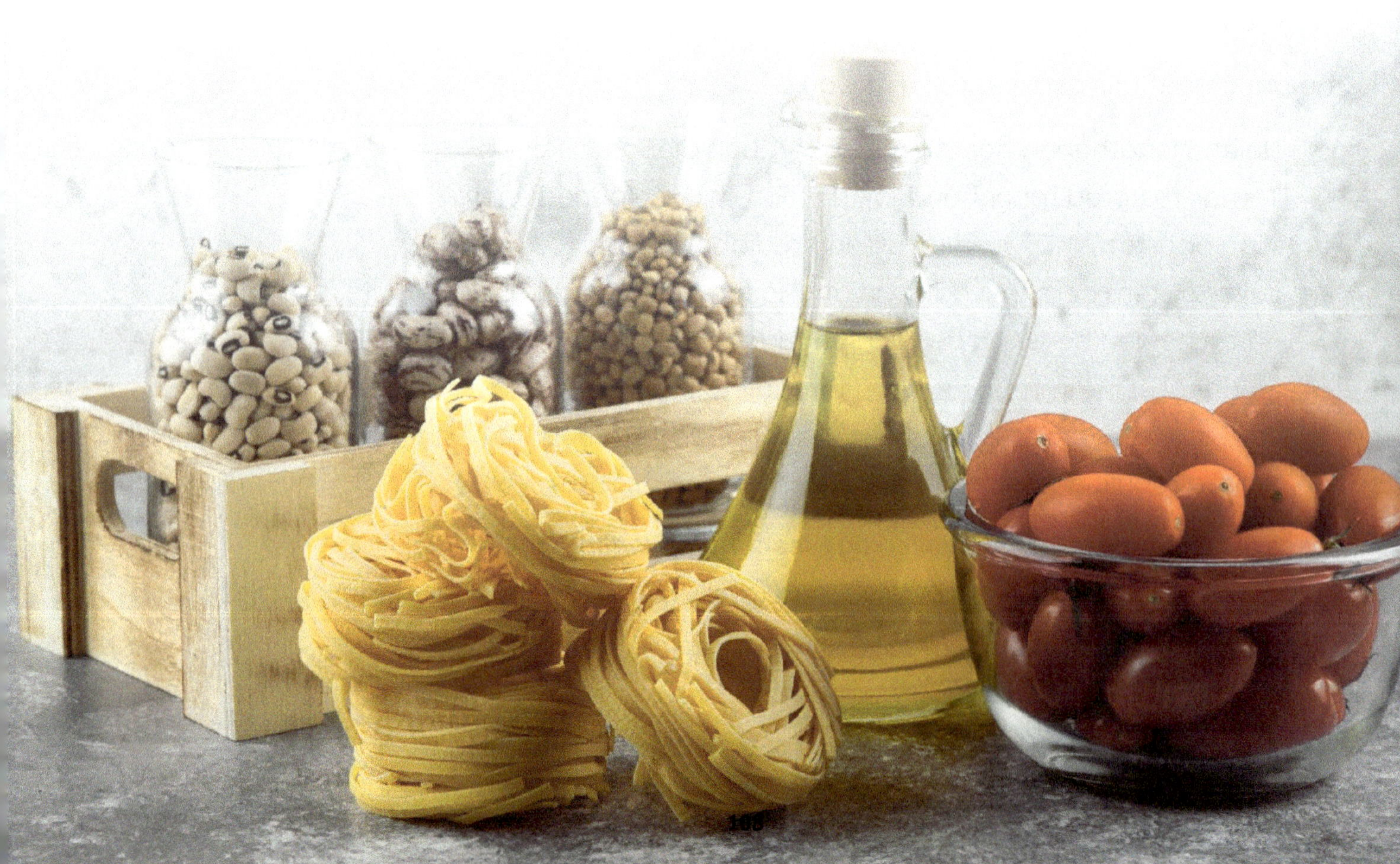

CHAPTER 5
Peak Performance

The Pursuit of Human Potential

When people think of athletes, they think of speed, power, and glory. When they think of performers—actors, dancers, musicians—they think of artistry and presence. Yet behind the spotlight lies the same challenge: the body and mind must work at extraordinary levels under immense pressure.

Nutrition, psychology, and exercise intersect here. For an athlete to push past fatigue or a performer to embody a character night after night, fuel is not optional. It is strategy.

Food becomes performance medicine. Exercise becomes both training and therapy.

Psychology, resilience, focus, and recovery are the glue that holds it together.

This chapter explores the science of high performance through the lens of athletes, performers, and those battling internal challenges like ADHD and trauma. We will see how nutrition and exercise fuel resilience, how regenerative medicine supports recovery, and why coaches and nutritionists are essential allies.

Through case studies, journal data, and lived experiences, we will uncover the blueprint for thriving at the highest levels.

SECTION 1: NUTRITION AS PERFORMANCE MEDICINE

At the core of athletic and artistic excellence is energy. The body's demand for glucose, amino acids, fatty acids, and micronutrients is magnified under stress. Suboptimal nutrition leads to fatigue, injury, and burnout. Optimal nutrition fuels mastery.

The Evidence

- Performance and Whole Foods: International Journal of Sport Nutrition and Exercise Metabolism (2019): Athletes who consumed diets rich in whole foods had 25% lower injury rates and faster recovery times compared to those on processed diets.

- Anti-Inflammatory Benefits: British Journal of Sports Medicine (2020): High-antioxidant diets improved muscle repair and reduced inflammation after training.
- Protein Requirements: Journal of the International Society of Sports Nutrition (2018): Adequate protein intake (1.6-2.2 g/kg daily) is essential for performance and recovery. Athletes need significantly more protein than sedentary individuals.
- Carbohydrate Timing: Sports Medicine (2018): Strategic carbohydrate timing around training maximizes glycogen stores and improves endurance performance.

CASE STUDY: Elite Athletes and Plant-Based Eating

Serena Williams, one of the greatest athletes of all time, has spoken openly about using plant-based eating to recover and sustain energy. After injuries and postpartum challenges, she returned to competition with nutrition as a core strategy.

The Approach: Williams emphasized:

- Plant-forward meals rich in vegetables, legumes, whole grains
- Strategic protein timing for recovery
- Anti-inflammatory foods to support joint health
- Hydration protocols

She returned to elite competition, won major titles, and sustained her career into her 40s.

Research (2019): Plant-based athletes showed comparable or superior performance to omnivorous athletes when protein and nutrient needs were met. Anti-inflammatory benefits supported recovery and reduced injury risk.

The Lesson: Even at the highest levels of sport, food is as critical as training. Performance nutrition is not about one diet—it is about meeting individual needs with quality fuel.

SECTION 2: ADHD AND PERFORMANCE — FOCUS THROUGH FOOD AND EXERCISE

Athletes and professionals with ADHD face unique challenges. Impulsivity, distractibility, and inconsistent energy can derail performance. Yet with structured nutrition, hydration, and exercise, ADHD becomes a challenge that can be managed—and sometimes transformed into an advantage.

The Evidence

- Omega-3s for Attention: Nutrients (2020): Omega-3 fatty acids improved attention and reduced hyperactivity in ADHD patients. The effect was most pronounced in those with low baseline omega-3 in-take.

- Exercise and Executive Function: Journal of Attention Disorders (2018): Regular exercise improved executive function and reduced impulsivity in adults with ADHD. Cardiovascular exercise showed particular benefit.
- Protein and Dopamine: Harvard Health Review (2019): Protein-rich breakfasts provide amino acid precursors for dopamine synthesis, improving focus and reducing ADHD symptom fluctuation.
- Blood Sugar Stability: Stable blood sugar from balanced meals reduces the "crash-and-spike" pattern that worsens ADHD symptoms.

CASE STUDY: My ADHD Journey—Food, Focus, and the Final Exam

During my last step of medical licensure, I faced ADHD head-on. I had failed the exam five times. Each failure was devastating—not just academically, but existentially. Without passing, I could not practice medicine in the United States.

The Challenge: ADHD made sustained focus impossible. During exams, my mind wandered. I had read questions three times without comprehension. Time management collapsed under pressure.

The Intervention: On my sixth attempt, I finally sought comprehensive help:

Medication: Started proper ADHD medication (prescribed and monitored)

Nutrition:

- High-protein breakfasts: Eggs with spinach, Greek yogurt with nuts (dopamine precursors)
- Eliminated sugar: No refined carbs or sweets (prevented glucose crashes)
- Omega-3 supplementation: Fish oil 2,000mg daily
- Consistent hydration: Water bottle everywhere I went (dehydration worsens attention)
- Regular meals: No skipping, no long gaps (stable glucose = stable focus)

Exercise:

- Daily movement: 30-minute walks in the morning (cleared brain fog)
- Strength training: 3x/week (improved executive function)

Structure:

- Consistent sleep: 7-8 hours nightly, same bedtime
- Study in intervals: 25-minute focused blocks with 5-minute breaks

The Results

Exam Day: For the first time, my mind stayed present. I could read questions once and comprehend. Time management held. ***Final score: PASSED.***

Without that combination of medication, nutrition, hydration, and exercise, I would not be a physician in the United States today. That victory was not just academic—it was fueled by food, movement, and resilience.

The Science: My experience mirrors research: omega-3s improve attention (Nutrients, 2020), protein stabilizes focus, exercise enhances executive function (Journal of Attention Disorders, 2018), and hydration prevents cognitive decline.

The Lesson: ADHD is not a life sentence of struggle. With the right combination of medication, nutrition, and structure, focus returns. Performance becomes possible.

CASE STUDY: Jamal's Academic Breakthrough

Jamal, twenty-two, was a college student who had failed two classes despite taking ADHD medication. His diet revolved around energy drinks and late-night fast food. He described feeling "scattered, exhausted, and defeated."

The Challenge: Medication alone was not enough. His lifestyle undermined the medication's effectiveness.

The Intervention: We restructured his daily rhythm:

Nutrition:

- Protein-rich breakfasts: Scrambled eggs with vegetables (no more skipping breakfast)
- Omega-3 supplementation: Fish oil + salmon 2x/week
- Eliminated energy drinks: Replaced with water and green tea (steady caffeine, no crash)
- Vegetables with every meal: Spinach, broccoli, peppers (micronutrients for brain function)
- Consistent meal timing: Three meals, two snacks, no long gaps

Exercise:

- Morning walks: 20 minutes before first class
- Gym 3x/week: Strength training and basketball

Study habits:

- Pomodoro technique: 25-minute focus blocks
- Accountability partner: Study group 3x/week

The Results

Month 1: Focus during lectures noticeably improved

Month 3: Energy steady throughout the day, no afternoon crashes Semester end: Passed both classes with B+ grades

Quote: "If I hadn't changed my food and added exercise, medication alone wouldn't have been enough. Now I actually feel like I can succeed."

The Science: Jamal's success reflects meta-analyses showing omega-3s, protein, and exercise improve ADHD symptoms when combined with medication.

The Lesson: Medication opens the door. Nutrition and exercise walk you through it.

SECTION 3: TRAUMA, RESILIENCE, AND PERFORMANCE

Trauma—whether physical injury or emotional experience—leaves deep imprints. For athletes, trauma might come from career-ending injuries or subjective experiences. For performers, trauma may manifest in anxiety, eating disorders, or substance use.

Nutrition and exercise serve as part of the recovery process.

The Evidence

- Trauma and Inflammation: Frontiers in Psychology (2020): Trauma survivors had 60% higher rates of obesity and disordered eating, but anti-inflammatory diets reduced cortisol and improved resilience.
- Exercise and PTSD: Journal of Psychiatric Research (2019): Exercise-based interventions reduced PTSD symptoms by 35%. Cardio-vascular exercise and strength training both showed benefit.
- Omega-3s and Emotional Regulation: Neuroscience & Biobehavioral Reviews (2018): Omega-3 supplementation improved emotional regulation in trauma survivors by reducing neuroinflammation.

CASE STUDY: Michael Phelps and Mental Health

Olympic swimmer Michael Phelps has been candid about his struggles with depression, anxiety, and suicidal thoughts. His battles came despite—or perhaps because of—his extraordinary athletic success.

The Challenge: Performance pressure, post-Olympic depression, and unaddressed trauma created a mental health crisis.

The Approach: Phelps' recovery involved:

- Therapy: Regular sessions with mental health professionals

- Medication: When needed, responsibly managed
- Structured lifestyle: Training, nutrition, sleep hygiene
- Nutrition focus: Whole foods, anti-inflammatory eating, hydration
- Community: Opening to family, teammates, and the public

The Results

Phelps not only recovered but became an advocate for mental health awareness in athletics. He returned to competition and won more Olympic medals.

The Science: Phelps' journey reflects research showing that elite performance requires mental health support. Nutrition, therapy, and exercise work together—not separately.

The Lesson: Performance is as much mental as physical, and both are deeply shaped by nutrition and lifestyle. Even the greatest athletes need comprehensive support.

SECTION 4: THE ROLE OF COACHES AND NUTRITIONISTS

At elite levels, self-discipline is not enough. Athletes and performers rely on coaches, trainers, and nutritionists to map out programs, correct form, and build accountability.

Why Coaches Matter

- Form Correction: Prevents injury in strength training and maximizes results
- Program Design: Tailors training to goals, balancing strength, endurance, and recovery
- Psychological Support: Coaches serve as motivators, mentors, and stabilizers
- Accountability: Keeps athletes consistent when motivation wanes

Why Nutritionists Matter

- Precision Fueling: Balances macronutrients for performance windows (pre-workout, post-workout, competition day)
- Recovery Planning: Designs meals to reduce inflammation and optimize repair
- Supplement Guidance: Determines what is evidence-based vs. marketing hype
- Longevity Focus: Guides athletes to sustain careers and health beyond competition

CASE STUDY: LeBron James and Longevity Investment

LeBron James, still performing at elite levels well into his late 30s (now 41), invests over $1 million annually in his body—coaches, trainers, nutritionists, recovery protocols, and medical support.

The Approach

- Customized nutrition: Diets tailored to his metabolic needs, training load, and recovery
- Recovery protocols: Cryotherapy, compression therapy, sleep optimization
- Strength and conditioning: Personalized programs that evolve with age
- Medical team: Ongoing monitoring, injury prevention, regenerative treatments

The Results:

At an age when most players have retired, LeBron continues to compete at the highest level. He has extended his career by over a decade compared to average NBA longevity.

The Lesson: Elite performance is not just talent—it is infrastructure. Coaches, nutritionists, and support teams extend careers and enhance resilience.

SECTION 5: REGENERATIVE MEDICINE IN PERFORMANCE

Regenerative medicine is transforming recovery for athletes and performers. From stem cell injections to platelet-rich plasma (PRP) therapy, these interventions reduce downtime and accelerate healing.

But nutrition is always the foundation.

The Evidence

- PRP Therapy: American Journal of Sports Medicine (2018): PRP therapy reduced recovery time in tendon injuries by 30%.
- Stem Cells and Nutrition: Journal of Stem Cell Research (2019): Nutritional status determined the success of stem cell therapies for joint injuries. Anti-inflammatory diets improved outcomes.
- Recovery Nutrition: Sports Health (2021): Regenerative medicine combined with anti-inflammatory diets improved long-term outcomes in musculoskeletal injuries.

CASE STUDY: Tiger Woods and Regeneration

Tiger Woods famously used platelet-rich plasma (PRP) therapy and stem cell treatments to recover from injuries that could have ended his career—multiple back surgeries, knee problems, and a severe car accident.

The Approach

- PRP injections: To accelerate tendon and ligament healing
- Stem cell therapy: For joint regeneration
- Disciplined nutrition: Anti-inflammatory diet to support healing environment
- Training modifications: Adapted golf swing to reduce stress on injured areas
- Sleep and recovery: Prioritized rest and regeneration

The Results:

Woods returned to competitive play and won the 2019 Masters—one of the greatest comebacks in sports history.

The Science: Tiger's recovery highlights the synergy between regenerative medicine and nutrition. Stem cells and PRP work best when the body is nutritionally prepared.

The Lesson: Cutting-edge therapies need old-fashioned nutrition to succeed.

SECTION 6: PERFORMERS AND ACTORS — NUTRITION UNDER PRESSURE

Actors, dancers, and musicians endure grueling schedules, irregular meals, and extreme physical demands. Nutrition becomes critical for energy, immunity, and mental clarity.

The Demands

- Long hours: 12-16 hour days on set or stage
- Physical transformations: Rapid weight gain/loss for roles
- Mental focus: Memorization, emotional intensity
- Sleep disruption: Early call times, night shoots
- Immune stress: Travel, close quarters, variable conditions

CASE STUDY: Hugh Jackman's Wolverine Transformation

Hugh Jackman famously transformed his physique for the Wolverine roles through extreme but structured nutrition and training.

The Approach

- High-protein diet: Lean meats, fish, eggs (muscle building)
- Strategic carbohydrates: Timing around workouts for energy and recovery
- Intermittent fasting: 16:8 pattern to maintain lean mass while cutting body fat
- Hydration protocols: Dehydration before shirtless scenes (short-term only)
- Professional guidance: Nutritionist and trainer oversight throughout

The Challenge: Maintaining muscle mass while reducing body fat to incredibly low levels—demanding and unsustainable long-term.

The Results:

Achieved the iconic physique multiple times across different films. Jackman has spoken about the discipline required and the unsustainability of maintaining that look year-round.

The Science: Jackman's approach reflects Journal of the International Society of Sports Nutrition (2018): high protein intake (2+ g/kg), strategic carb timing, and professional guidance allow for dramatic body transformations—but require careful monitoring.

The Lesson: Extreme transformations require extreme structure and professional oversight. The public should not attempt these without guidance.

CASE STUDY: Professional Dancers and Sustained Energy

Dancers at companies like the New York City Ballet perform 6-8 shows per week while rehearsing new works daily. Energy demands are massive, injury risk is high, and career longevity depends on nutrition.

The Approach: Dancers report that maintaining energy and preventing injury depends on:

- Plant-rich diets: Vegetables, fruits, whole grains for sustained energy
- Lean protein: For muscle repair without feeling heavy
- Hydration: Constant water intake (sweating during performances)
- Anti-inflammatory foods: Berries, olive oil, fish to protect joints
- Recovery nutrition: Post-performance meals with protein and carbs

The Challenge: Balancing enough food for energy demands while maintaining the physique required for ballet.

Dancers who prioritize nutrition report fewer injuries, sustained energy across performances, and longer careers.

The Lesson: Performers are athletes too. Nutrition determines whether they can sustain excellence or burn out.

SECTION 7: EXERCISE AS MEDICINE

Nutrition and psychology intersect most powerfully in exercise. Beyond strength and endurance, exercise transforms brain chemistry, enhances resilience, and builds confidence.

The Evidence

Mental Health Benefits

- Lancet Psychiatry (2019): Exercise reduced depression symptoms by 43% compared to no intervention.

Anxiety Reduction

- JAMA Psychiatry (2018): Regular exercise lowered the risk of anxiety disorders by 26%.

ADHD and Executive Function

- Sports Medicine (2020): Resistance training improved executive function in ADHD patients.

Neuroplasticity

- Nature Neuroscience (2017): Exercise increases brain-derived neurotrophic factor (BDNF), supporting neuroplasticity and cognitive resilience.

Types of Exercise for Performance

Pilates

- Enhances core strength and body awareness
- Reduces anxiety and improves posture
- Popular among dancers, actors, and those recovering from injury

Strength Training

- Builds muscle, improves dopamine regulation
- Essential for ADHD symptom management
- Supports bone density and metabolic health

Aerobic Exercise

- Enhances cardiovascular health
- Boosts serotonin and reduces trauma-related stress
- Improves endurance and stamina

Flexibility Work (Yoga, Stretching)

- Prevents injury
- Reduces cortisol
- Improves mind-body connection

SECTION 8: THE 7-DAY HIGH-PERFORMANCE PLAN

GOAL: Maximize physical performance, mental focus, and recovery FOCUS: Strategic protein timing, anti-inflammatory foods, hydration, exercise integration

DAY 1: POWER FOUNDATION

MORNING

Pre-Workout: Banana + almond butter (quick energy, no GI distress) Post-Workout Breakfast: Scrambled eggs + spinach + sweet potato + olive oil

Why: Protein for muscle repair, complex carbs replenish glycogen, anti-inflammatory fats

MIDDAY

High-Protein Lunch: Grilled chicken + quinoa + roasted vegetables + olive oil Why: Sustained energy, complete protein, antioxidants for recovery

EVENING

Recovery Dinner: Salmon + brown rice + steamed broccoli Why: Omega-3s reduce inflammation, carbs restore glycogen, cruciferous vegetables support detox

EXERCISE: Strength training (45 min), focus on major muscle groups

HYDRATION: 3+ liters water, electrolytes if sweating heavily

DAY 2: ENDURANCE SUPPORT

MORNING

Pre-Workout: Oatmeal + berries + walnuts

Why: Slow-digesting carbs for sustained energy

Post-Workout: Greek yogurt + honey + chia seeds Why: Protein + quick carbs for glycogen replenishment

MIDDAY

Lunch: Lentil soup + whole grain bread + side salad Why: Plant protein, fiber, sustained energy without heaviness

EVENING

Dinner: Turkey + roasted sweet potatoes + Brussels sprouts

Why: Lean protein, complex carbs, anti-inflammatory cruciferous vegetables

EXERCISE: Cardiovascular training (60 min moderate intensity)

PRACTICE: Visualization exercise before bed (mental performance prep)

DAY 3: RECOVERY & REPAIR

MORNING

Breakfast: Smoothie (kefir + banana + spinach + protein powder + flaxseed) Why: Probiotics, easy-to-digest protein, anti-inflammatory omega-3s

MIDDAY

Lunch: Mediterranean grain bowl (quinoa + chickpeas + vegetables + olive oil + lemon)

Why: Complete nutrition, anti-inflammatory, promotes tissue repair

EVENING

Dinner: Cod + mashed cauliflower + sautéed kale

Why: Lean protein, low-inflammatory vegetables, easy to digest

EXERCISE: Active recovery (30 min walk or gentle yoga)

PRACTICE: Foam rolling, stretching (15 min)

DAY 4: FOCUS & PRECISION

MORNING

Pre-Workout: Apple + almond butter

Post-Workout: Eggs + avocado + whole grain toast

Why: Healthy fats support brain function, protein aids recovery

MIDDAY

Lunch: Salmon salad (greens + salmon + walnuts + olive oil + lemon) Why: Omega-3s for cognitive function and inflammation control

EVENING

Dinner: Grass-fed beef (small portion) + roasted vegetables + quinoa Why: Iron and zinc for cognitive function, complete nutrition

EXERCISE: Skill work or sport-specific training (60 min)

PRACTICE: Mental focus drills, mindfulness (10 min)

DAY 5: ANTI-INFLAMMATORY EMPHASIS MORNING

Breakfast: Turmeric lentil bowl + spinach + poached egg

Why: Curcumin reduces inflammation, protein supports recovery

MIDDAY

Lunch: Chickpea turmeric stew + side salad

Why: Plant protein, anti-inflammatory spices, easy to digest

EVENING

Dinner: Grilled sardines + arugula + roasted peppers + olive oil Why: Maximum omega-3s, polyphenols, antioxidants

EXERCISE: Pilates or yoga (60 min)

PRACTICE: Gratitude journaling (performance psychology)

DAY 6: PEAK PERFORMANCE PREP

MORNING

Pre-Competition: Oatmeal + banana + honey (3 hours before) Why: Easily digestible carbs for maximum glycogen

During Competition: Electrolyte drink, energy gels if needed

Post-Competition: Chocolate milk or recovery shake (protein + carbs within 30 min)

Why: Rapid glycogen replenishment, muscle repair initiation

EVENING

Recovery Dinner: Salmon + sweet potato + steamed vegetables Why: Complete recovery nutrition

EXERCISE: Competition or peak performance event

PRACTICE: Post-performance reflection and notes

DAY 7: RESTORATION

MORNING

Breakfast: Chia pudding + berries + walnuts Why: Omega-3s, antioxidants, gentle on digestive system

MIDDAY

Lunch: Bone broth + vegetables + whole grain bread Why: Collagen for tissue repair, easy to digest, restorative

EVENING

Dinner: Light vegetable curry + brown rice Why: Anti-inflammatory spices, plant-based recovery

EXERCISE: Complete rest or exceptionally light movement (20 min walk)

PRACTICE: Reflect on week, set next week's goals, sleep 9+ hours

CLOSING: EXCELLENCE IS A CHOICE

Athletes, performers, and high achievers prove one thing: excellence is not luck. It is the daily discipline of eating well, training consistently, and mastering psychology.

We have seen:

- Serena Williams, LeBron James, Tiger Woods harness nutrition, and regenerative medicine
- Hugh Jackman and professional dancers sustain demanding careers through strategic nutrition
- Michael Phelps demonstrate that mental health requires comprehensive support
- My own ADHD journey and Jamal's breakthrough show that focus returns when nutrition partners with medication
- Coaches and nutritionists extend careers and maximize performance

But just as importantly, we have seen ordinary people achieve extraordinary results:

- Students passing exams they had failed multiple times
- Trauma survivors reclaiming resilience
- Professionals managing ADHD through food and movement

Peak performances are not reserved for Olympic athletes. It is available to anyone who chooses to fuel themselves properly, move consistently, and support their mental health.

Your peak performance may not be on a court or a stage, but in your daily life—your work, your relationships, your ability to show up fully present.

Fuel yourself like an athlete.

Train yourself as a performer.

Nourish your mind like a healer.

Because peak performance is not about being the best in the world. It is about being the best version of yourself.

And that begins with what you put on your plate, how you move your body, and how you support your mind. **One meal, one practice, one day at a time.**

CHAPTER 6
The Roadmap to Regeneration

Living the Future Today

We have reached a turning point in medicine. For decades, the conversation was about survival—preventing heart attacks, managing diabetes, prolonging life after a cancer diagnosis. But the new era is about more: it is about reversal, regeneration, and thriving.

Food, exercise, therapy, regenerative medicine, and psychiatry are not silos. They are interwoven into a single truth: change your diet, change your mind, change your life.

This concluding chapter is not about more statistics or more studies—though we will ground the message in data. It is about the possibility. About building a roadmap you can live by every day, about showing you that no matter your starting point, you have the power to create a future of resilience, energy, and grace.

THE CORE PRINCIPLES OF TRANSFORMATION

Through all science, case studies, diets, fasting, supplements, and certain principles rise to the surface. These are the non-negotiables of longevity and health.

Principle 1: Food as Medicine

Every bite is either pro-inflammatory or anti-inflammatory. Every meal builds disease or builds health.

The research is unambiguous:

- Mediterranean diet reduces cardiovascular risk by 30% (NEJM, 2013)
- Plant-based eating reverses diabetes in up to 46% of patients (Diabetes Care, 2017)
- MIND diet reduces Alzheimer's risk by 53% (Alzheimer's & Dementia, 2015)

- Diet improves depression remission by 32% (SMILES Trial, 2017) Food is not a side note. It is the main story.

Principle 2: Movement as Therapy

Exercise is not a punishment. It is a prescription for mood, resilience, and cognitive protection.

The evidence:

- Exercise reduces depression by 43% (Lancet Psychiatry, 2019)
- Physical activity lowers anxiety disorder risk by 26% (JAMA Psychiatry, 2018)
- Strength training improves executive function in ADHD (Sports Medicine, 2020)
- Regular movement increases BDNF (brain-derived neurotrophic factor), supporting neuroplasticity

Movement is medicine. Daily.

Principle 3: Psychiatry as Partnership

Medications, when needed, are lifesaving. But their effect is magnified when combined with nutrition and therapy.

Throughout this book, we have seen:

- Elena's depression lifted when food gave her medication something to work with
- My own ADHD became manageable when nutrition partnered with medication
- Michael's bipolar disorder stabilized with structured meals alongside medication

Medication is not a weakness. It is a tool. And tools work better with the right foundation.

Principle 4: Regeneration as Mindset

Aging is not declining. It is an adaptation. With fasting, peptides, NAD+, and lifestyle, the body regenerates.

We have seen:

- Helena lengthening her telomeres through diet and stress management
- Tomas restoring mitochondrial function and reclaiming energy
- Alan boosting NAD+ and reversing prediabetes
- Ethan resetting his immune system through fasting

Biological age can be slowed—and in some measures, reversed.

Principle 5: Connection as Medicine

Longevity is not only about the body. Community, love, and purpose extend lifespan as much as diet.

Blue Zones research confirms:

- Social connection reduces mortality risk by 50% (PLOS Medicine, 2010)
- Purpose (Ikigai in Okinawa) correlates with 7+ years longer lifespan
- Eating with others improves dietary quality and mental health

Isolation kills. Connection heals.

STORIES THAT PROVE CHANGE IS POSSIBLE

Throughout this book, you have met people whose lives transformed:

1. My husband reversed hypertension in three months at age 45, without medication, simply changing his diet.
2. Lisa sent type 2 diabetes into remission, came off insulin, and lost 30 pounds.
3. Michael lifted his depression when Mediterranean eating partnered with therapy and medication.
4. Sofia has still been cancer-free for 10 years through cruciferous vegetables, flaxseed, and movement.
5. Samuel's heart disease reversed with olive oil, beans, and exercise—his cardiologist reduced medications.
6. Rosa breathed easier with COPD through antioxidants and omega-3s.
7. Elena reclaimed her mood when food gave her antidepressants a foundation to work on.
8. Hannah's anxiety calmed when stable glucose and magnesium lowered her nervous system's alarm.
9. Jamal passed his classes when omega-3s and protein partnered with ADHD medication.
10. Helena lengthened her telomeres and reversed biological aging markers.
11. Tomas defeated chronic fatigue by restoring mitochondrial function.
12. Alan boosted NAD+ and turned back his metabolic clock.

Each story proves what journals confirm: food is medicine. And medicine is food.

THE DATA: THE EVIDENCE OF CHANGE

Let us anchor these stories in the numbers:

1. Global Burden of Disease Study (Lancet, 2019): Poor diet accounts for 11 million deaths annually, more than smoking, alcohol, or inactivity combined.
2. American Heart Association: 80% of cardiovascular disease is preventable through lifestyle.
3. World Health Organization: 70% of premature deaths globally are lifestyle driven.
4. Harvard School of Public Health: Mediterranean diet reduces cardiovascular risk by 30%.
5. SMILES Trial: Mediterranean diet improved depression remission by 32%.
6. Diabetes Prevention Program: Lifestyle changes reduced diabetes incidence by 58%—twice as effective as metformin.
7. World Cancer Research Fund: 30-50% of cancers are preventable through diet and lifestyle.
8. CDC (2022): 90% of U.S. healthcare spending goes to chronic diseases, most of which are preventable.
9. American Journal of Lifestyle Medicine (2020): Plant-based diets reduced medication costs by 29% within one year.
10. American Heart Association: Every $1 invested in prevention saves $3 in future medical costs.

This is no longer a debate. It is a fact.

THE ROADMAP: YOUR PERSONAL PLAN

This roadmap is not abstract. It is practical, daily, and actionable.

Step 1: Redefine food

See food not as calories, but as information.

Ask yourself: "Will this meal reduce inflammation or increase it?" Choose anti-inflammatory foods:

Vegetables (especially leafy greens and cruciferous)

- Beans and lentils
- Olive oil
- Fish (salmon, sardines)
- Nuts and seeds
- Berries

- Whole grains

Limit:

- Processed foods
- Refined sugars
- Trans fats
- Excessive red meat
- Ultra-processed snacks

Step 2: Move Every Day

Make movement non-negotiable.

Minimum daily commitment:

- 30-minute walk (or equivalent)
- Strength training 2x/week
- Flexibility work (yoga, Pilates, stretching) 1-2x/week

Why it matters:

- Reduces depression and anxiety
- Improves insulin sensitivity
- Increases BDNF (brain growth factor)
- Supports cardiovascular health
- Enhances sleep quality

Exercise is the second half of nutrition—together they form the foundation of health.

Step 3: Fast Wisely

Adopt time-restricted eating or periodic fasting.

Options:

- 12-14 hour overnight fast: Finish dinner by 7 PM, breakfast at 9 AM (easiest entry point)
- 16:8 intermittent fasting: 16 hours fasting, 8-hour eating window
- 5:2 pattern: 5 days normal eating, 2 days reduced calories (500-600 calories)
- Fasting-mimicking diet: 5 days/month, 800-1,100 calories/day, plant-based (under medical supervision)

Benefits:

- Triggers autophagy (cellular cleanup)
- Increases stem cell production

- Boosts NAD+ levels
- Improves insulin sensitivity
- Reduces inflammation

Important: Consult with your physician before beginning any fasting protocol, especially if you have medical conditions or take medications.

Step 4: Support the Microbiome

Feed your gut bacteria—they feed you back.

Daily microbiome support:

- Fermented foods: Kefir, yogurt, sauerkraut, kimchi, miso
- Prebiotic fiber: Garlic, onions, asparagus, bananas, oats, beans
- Polyphenols: Berries, green tea, dark chocolate, olive oil
- Diverse vegetables: Aim for 30+ different plant foods per week

Why it matters:

- 70% of immune system lives in the gut
- Gut bacteria produce neurotransmitters (serotonin, dopamine precursors)
- Microbiome diversity correlates with longevity
- Gut-brain axis influences mood, cognition, and behavior

Step 5: Embrace Regenerative Tools

With medical guidance, consider:

Supplements:

- Omega-3s: 1,000-2,000mg EPA+DHA daily
- Vitamin D: 1,000-2,000 IU daily (test levels first)
- Curcumin: 500-1,000mg with black pepper (enhances absorption)
- NAD+ precursors: NMN or NR (emerging research, physician guidance recommended)
- Magnesium: 300-400mg daily (especially for anxiety, sleep, muscle recovery)

Advanced interventions (with physician oversight):

- Peptides: BPC-157, Thymosin Alpha-1 (for specific healing needs)
- Stem cell therapies: For joint injuries, tissue regeneration
- Precision nutrition tools: Continuous glucose monitors, microbiome testing

Remember: Supplements supplement. They do not replace whole food.

Step 6: Integrate Mental Health

If you suffer from depression, anxiety, ADHD, bipolar disorder, trauma, or other mental health challenges, know that psychiatry plus nutrition is more powerful than either alone.

What works:

- Medication when needed: Not weakness, but tool
- Therapy: CBT, trauma-informed therapy, mindfulness-based approaches
- Nutrition: Anti-inflammatory eating, stable glucose, omega-3s, probiotics
- Exercise: Proven to reduce symptoms across all psychiatric conditions
- Sleep: 7-8 hours nightly, consistent schedule
- Social connection: Reduces isolation, improves outcomes

Medications are not crutches—they are bridges. And nutrition strengthens those bridges.

Step 7: Connection and Purpose

Eat with others. Share meals with your family. Pursue purpose.

Blue Zones data shows that community and meaning are as important as diet:

- Okinawans have "Ikigai" (reason for being)
- Sardinians eat together, multiple generations at the table
- Adventists in Loma Linda prioritize Sabbath and community
- Ikarians gather daily in village squares

Practical applications:

- Cook with others: Involve family, friends, or join cooking classes
- Eat together: At least one shared meal daily
- Volunteer: Purpose extends lifespan
- Join groups: Walking clubs, book clubs, faith communities

Isolation is a risk factor as deadly as smoking. Connection is a protective medicine.

Step 8: Build Longevity Identity

Shift your mindset: "I am someone who eats and lives for resilience." Identity-based habits are more powerful than goal-based habits.

Instead of: "I want to lose 20 pounds" (goal-based, temporary) **Say:** "I am someone who nourishes my body with whole foods" (identity-based, permanent)

Examples:

- "I am someone who walks daily"
- "I am someone who eats vegetables at every meal"

- "I am someone who prioritizes sleep"
- "I am someone who manages stress through movement"

Anchor your habits to identity, not willpower. Identity endures when motivation fades.

THE 30-DAY IMPLEMENTATION ROADMAP

This is your practical, step-by-step guide to transformation.

WEEK 1: RESET

Focus: Remove obstacles, set up foundation

Actions:

- Clear the pantry:
  - Remove processed foods, refined sugars, trans fats
  - Stock essentials: beans, olive oil, whole grains, nuts, frozen vegetables
- Begin daily walks:
  - 30 minutes minimum
  - Morning preferred (sets tone for day)
- Start food journal:
  - Track what you eat
  - Note energy levels, mood, sleep
- Hydration baseline:
  - 8 glasses water daily minimum
  - Lemon water in morning
- Sleep hygiene:
  - Consistent bedtime
  - 7-8 hours nightly
  - No screens 1 hour before bed

Sample Day:

- Morning: Oatmeal + blueberries + walnuts, walk 30 min
- Midday: Lentil soup + whole grain bread, water
- Evening: Salmon + roasted vegetables + quinoa
- Practice: Journal emotions and energy levels

WEEK 2: REBUILD

Focus: Add structure, increase movement

Actions:

- Add beans daily:
  - Breakfast, lunch, or dinner
  - Batch-cook on Sundays
- Start strength training:
  - Bodyweight exercises or gym
  - 2x this week, 20-30 minutes
- Begin 12-hour overnight fast:
  - Finish dinner by 7 PM
  - Breakfast at 7 AM or later
- Add fermented foods:
  - Kefir, yogurt, or sauerkraut daily
- Meal prep Sunday:
  - Cook grains, beans, roast vegetables
  - Prep for the week

Sample Day:

- Morning: Greek yogurt + berries + almonds, strength training 30 min
- Midday: Black bean bowl + avocado + vegetables
- Evening: Grilled chicken + Brussels sprouts + barley
- Practice: 12-hour fast (dinner by 7 PM)

WEEK 3: REGENERATE

Focus: Improve, introduce advanced strategies

Actions:

- Extend fasting window:
  - Try 14-16 hours (finish dinner by 6 PM, breakfast at 10 AM)
  - 3-4 days this week
- Add omega-3 supplementation:
  - 1,000-2,000mg EPA+DHA
  - Or increase fish to 3-4x/week
- Daily meditation:
  - 5-10 minutes
  - Morning or before bed
- Increase vegetables:
  - Aim for 7-9 servings daily
  - Half your plate at lunch and dinner

- Social eating:
    - Share at least 3 meals with others this week

Sample Day:

- Morning: 16-hour fast completes, smoothie (kefir + spinach + berries + chia)
- Midday: Mediterranean grain bowl + olive oil
- Evening: Sardines + roasted vegetables + whole grain bread
- Practice: 10 min meditation, eat dinner with family

WEEK 4: REINFORCE

Focus: Make it sustainable, plan for long-term

Actions:

- Evaluate and adjust:
    - Review food journal
    - Note what worked, what did not
    - Find 3 habits to continue
- Blend exercise:
    - Aerobic 3x, strength 2x, flexibility 1x
    - Mix activities for sustainability
- Practice 80/20:
    - 80% whole foods, 20% flexibility
    - One treat meal weekly (mindfully enjoyed)
- Plan next month:
    - Set 3 specific goals
    - Schedule meal prep times
    - Book any needed appointments (doctor, nutritionist, therapist)
- Gratitude practice:
    - Daily journaling
    - Notice changes (sleep, energy, mood, weight)

Sample Day:

- Morning: Chia pudding + pomegranate + walnuts, Pilates 45 min
- Midday: Chickpea salad + vegetables + olive oil
- Evening: Salmon + sweet potato + kale
- Practice: Gratitude journal, reflect on 30-day progress

TROUBLESHOOTING COMMON OBSTACLES

"I don't have time to cook"

Solutions:

- Batch **PREP:** 90 minutes on Sunday feeds you all week
- One-pot meals: Soups, stews, sheet pan dinners (15 min prep, cook while you do other things)
- Frozen vegetables: Just as nutritious, zero prep
- Canned beans: Ready in seconds
- Meal delivery: Healthy options like prepared meal services (invest in health)

"Healthy food is expensive"

Reality check:

- Beans, lentils, oats, rice, frozen vegetables are cheaper than processed foods
- Medical bills are more expensive than groceries
- Prevention saves money long-term

Budget strategies:

- Buy in bulk (beans, grains, nuts)
- Frozen > fresh if budget is tight
- Seasonal produce
- Skip expensive "superfoods"—regular vegetables work just as well
- Cook at home vs. eating out

"My family won't eat this way"

Solutions:

- Start with what they will accept: Add vegetables to familiar dishes
- Cook once, customize: Base meal + individual add-ons
- Lead by example: Your health transformation will inspire
- Include them: Kids who cook eat better
- Do not force: Offer options, model healthy eating

"I travel constantly for work"

Solutions:

- Airport/hotel hacks: Salads, grilled fish, oatmeal, fruit
- Pack snacks: Nuts, protein bars, apples
- Request: Hotel room with mini-fridge or kitchenette
- Research: Healthy restaurants near hotel
- Hydration: Carry refillable water bottle

- Exercise: Bodyweight workouts in hotel room, walk instead of taxi when possible

"I have food allergies/intolerances"

Solutions:

- Gluten-free: Quinoa, rice, oats (certified GF), beans, vegetables
- Dairy-free: Almond milk, coconut yogurt, nutritional yeast
- Nut allergies: Seeds (sunflower, pumpkin, chia, hemp), tahini
- Work with: Registered dietitian to ensure nutrient adequacy
- Focus on: What you CAN eat, not restrictions

"I've tried before and failed"

Reframe:

- Earlier attempts were learning experiences, not failures
- You are different now—you have better information, better support
- Start smaller: One meal, one day, one week
- Progress > perfection: 80% consistency beats 100% for 3 days then quitting
- Get support: Doctor, nutritionist, therapist, cooking class, accountability partner

THE ECONOMICS OF PREVENTION

Prevention is not only about adding years to life. It saves money.

The Data:

- CDC (2022): 90% of U.S. healthcare spending goes to chronic diseases, most preventable through lifestyle.
- American Journal of Lifestyle Medicine (2020): Patients adopting plant-based diets reduced medication costs by 29% within one year.
- American Heart Association: Every $1 invested in preventive lifestyle changes saves $3 in future medical costs.

Hidden costs of chronic disease:

- Medications: $200-500+/month for multiple prescriptions
- Doctor visits: Copays, specialists, tests
- Lost productivity: Sick days, reduced capacity
- Reduced quality of life: Priceless

Investment in prevention:

- Whole foods: Budget-friendly when you buy smart
- Exercise: Free (walking) or minimal (gym membership)
- Sleep: Free

- Stress management: Free (meditation apps, walking, journaling)

Prevention is not only health care. It is financial freedom.

THE PSYCHOLOGY OF COMMITMENT

Behavior change requires more than knowledge. It requires a mindset.

Identity Shift

Instead of: "I'm on a diet" (temporary, external)

Say: "I am someone who nourishes my body" (permanent, internal)

Health Psychology (2017): Patients who shifted to identity-based health habits were twice as likely to sustain changes in one year.

Micro-Wins Matter

Celebrate minor changes:

- Slept through the night for the first time in months
- Walked 30 minutes daily for a week
- Chose water over soda 5 days straight
- Cooked dinner 3 nights instead of takeout

Small wins build momentum. Perfection creates pressure that leads to failure.

Accountability

Work with professionals:

- Physician: Monitors health markers, prescribes medications if needed
- Nutritionist/Dietitian: Personalizes nutrition plans
- Therapist: Addresses emotional eating, trauma, mental health
- Psychiatrist: Manages medication for mental health conditions
- Coach/Trainer: Guides exercise, prevents injury
- Community: Support groups, cooking classes, walking clubs

You do not have to do this alone. In fact, you should not.

Purpose

Anchor habits to what matters:

- "I want to see my grandchildren grow up"
- "I want to feel energetic, not exhausted"
- "I want to model health for my children"

- "I want to travel without mobility limitations"
- "I want to avoid my parents' health struggles"

Purpose fuels consistency when motivation fades.

MOTIVATIONAL CLOSING: IF I CAN, YOU CAN

I was a child who gave up sugar at 14 after learning it ages the body. I exercised through medical school in Brazil while my classmates lived on caffeine and junk food. I fought through ADHD, through exhaustion, through residency, and built resilience on food, hydration, and movement.

I watched my family members suffer from strokes, hypertension, and heart disease. I saw what happens when prevention is ignored. And I chose a different path.

My husband resisted my way of eating until his blood pressure rose to 180/95. Then he changed. Within months, his health rebounded. If he can, anyone can.

Lisa reversed diabetes. Michael lifted depression. Sofia defended against cancer.

Nadia healed from trauma.

Samuel reversed heart disease. Elena reclaimed her mood. Hannah calmed anxiety.

Jamal passed his exams.

Helena lengthened her telomeres. Tomas defeated fatigue.

Alan reversed his metabolic age.

This is the message: Food changes lives. Food prevents. Food reverses. Food regenerates.

The future may bring stem cells, gene editing, and AI-guided diets. But the present brings beans, olive oil, berries, fish, nuts, meditation, movement, connection, and purpose.

If I can thrive with ADHD...

If my husband can reverse hypertension...

If patients can overcome cancer, depression, diabetes, trauma, and fatigue... Then so can you.

YOUR ROADMAP BEGINS TODAY

You do not need perfection. You need one decision.

One meal that nourishes instead of inflames. One walk around the block.

One glass of water.

One conversation with your doctor

One night of good sleep

One moment of gratitude.

From that one decision, another follows. And another. Until you look back and realize:

You did not just change your diet. You changed your life.

The roadmap is clear. Science is proven.

The stories are real.

The only question left is: Will you begin? Change your diet, and you change your life.

Change your life, and you change the world around you.

The future begins now. On your plate. In your body. Through your choices.

Welcome to regeneration.

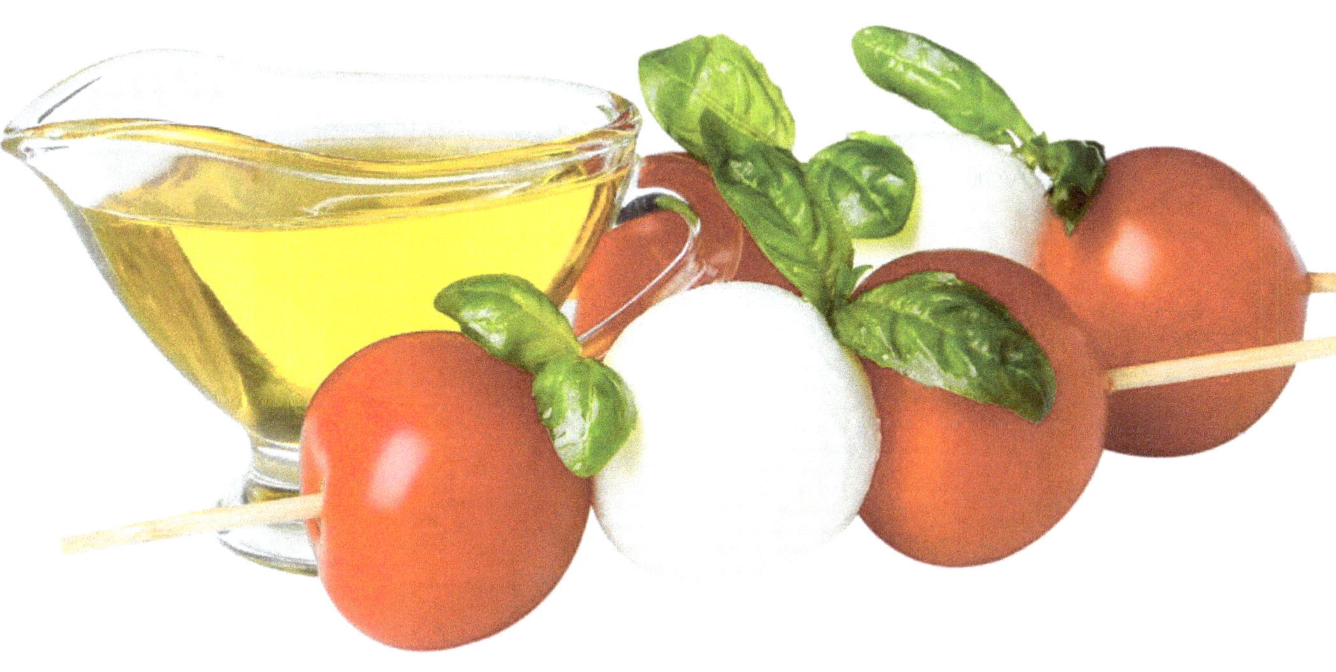

CHAPTER 7
Recipes for Life

A Complete Collection of Healing Meals

Food is not just sustenance—it is medicine, connection, and joy. This chapter brings together recipes designed to nourish every aspect of your health: cardiovascular protection, mental clarity, cancer prevention, anti-aging, performance, and recovery.

Each recipe is organized by purpose and meal type, making it easy to find exactly what you need. Whether you are seeking breakfast inspiration, quick lunches, healing dinners, or nourishing snacks, you will find clinically proven, delicious options here.

How to Use This Chapter:

- Browse by meal type: Find breakfast, lunch, dinner, or snacks
- Search by health goal: Look for tags like "Heart Health," "Mental Clarity," "Cancer Prevention"
- Start simple: Begin with 3-5 recipes you will make weekly
- Batch **PREP:** Many recipes are designed for meal prep and freezing
- Make it yours: Use variations to suit your taste and needs

Recipe 1: Overnight Oats with Omega-3 Power

Heart health • Mental clarity • Anti-aging

SERVES: 2 | **PREP:** 5 min + overnight | **COOK:** 0 min

WHY IT WORKS *This breakfast delivers soluble fiber from oats (lowers cholesterol), omega-3s from chia and walnuts (brain function), and anthocyanins from blueberries (memory protection). Perfect for busy mornings—prepare the night before.*

INGREDIENTS

Base:

- 1 cup rolled oats
- 2 tablespoons chia seeds
- 2 cups almond milk (or milk of choice)
- 1 teaspoon vanilla extract
- Pinch of salt

Toppings:

- 1 cup fresh or frozen blueberries
- ¼ cup chopped walnuts
- 1 tablespoon ground flaxseed
- Optional: 1 teaspoon honey or maple syrup per serving

METHOD

1. In a large jar or container, combine oats, chia seeds, milk, vanilla, and salt.
2. Stir well, ensuring no clumps.
3. Cover and refrigerate overnight (or minimum 4 hours).
4. In the morning, divide between two bowls.
5. Top each with blueberries, walnuts, and flaxseed.
6. Drizzle with honey if desired.

THE SCIENCE Oats have beta-glucan (lowers LDL cholesterol 5-10%, American Journal of Clinical Nutrition, 2014). Chia seeds provide 5g fiber and 2.5g omega-3s per tablespoon. Blueberries improve memory and protect neurons (Nutrients, 2020). Walnuts reduce cardiovascular mortality (Circulation, 2018).

NUTRITIONAL HIGHLIGHTS ~350 calories per serving | Rich in: Fiber (12g), Omega-3s (3g), Protein (10g), Antioxidants

VARIATIONS

- Chocolate version: Add 1 tablespoon cocoa powder
- Apple cinnamon: Replace blueberries with diced apple and cinnamon
- Protein boost: Stir in 2 tablespoons Greek yogurt or protein powder
- Savory: Skip sweet toppings, add hemp seeds and a drizzle of olive oil

STORAGE Prepare up to 5 servings in individual jars. Refrigerate up to 5 days. Add fresh toppings each morning.

Recipe 2: Mediterranean Veggie Scramble

ADHD focus • Energy • Heart health

SERVES: 2 | **PREP:** 5 min | **COOK:** 10 min

WHY IT WORKS *Eggs provide choline (acetylcholine production for memory and focus). Spinach delivers folate (reduces depression risk). Tomatoes add lycopene (cardiovascular protection). Perfect protein-rich breakfast for sustained energy and attention.*

INGREDIENTS

- 4 large eggs
- 2 cups fresh spinach
- ½ cup cherry tomatoes, halved
- ¼ cup diced red bell pepper
- ¼ cup crumbled feta (optional)
- 2 tablespoons extra virgin olive oil
- 2 garlic cloves, minced
- Salt and pepper to taste
- Fresh basil or parsley for garnish

METHOD

1. Heat 1 tablespoon olive oil in a large skillet over medium heat.
2. Add garlic, bell pepper, and tomatoes. Sauté for 3 minutes until softened.
3. Add spinach and cook until wilted (1-2 minutes).
4. In a bowl, whisk eggs with salt and pepper.
5. Push vegetables to the side of the pan, add remaining olive oil to the center.
6. Pour in eggs and scramble gently, incorporating vegetables as eggs cook.
7. Remove from heat when eggs are just set (still slightly creamy).
8. Top with feta if using, and fresh herbs.

THE SCIENCE Eggs supply choline for focus and memory. Spinach provides folate (deficiency linked to depression). Tomatoes deliver lycopene (reduces prostate cancer risk 20%, Cancer Epidemiology, 2016). Olive oil provides polyphenols for cardiovascular protection.

NUTRITIONAL HIGHLIGHTS ~280 calories per serving | Rich in: Protein (16g), Choline, Folate, Lycopene, Healthy fats

VARIATIONS

- Greek style: Add kalamata olives and oregano
- Mexican: Replace feta with avocado, add cumin and cilantro
- Vegan: Use scrambled tofu instead of eggs, nutritional yeast instead of feta
- Extra protein: Add white beans or chickpeas

STORAGE Best fresh. Can refrigerate scrambled eggs up to 2 days; reheat gently.

Recipe 3: Probiotic Power Smoothie

Gut-brain health • Mental clarity • Immune support

SERVES: 2 | **PREP:** 5 min | **COOK:** 0 min

WHY IT WORKS *Kefir provides diverse probiotics (gut-brain axis support). Spinach delivers magnesium (calms nervous system). Pumpkin seeds add zinc (immune function, mood regulation). Green tea provides L-theanine (smooths cortisol response). Perfect for busy mornings or post-work-out recovery.*

INGREDIENTS

- 1½ cups plain kefir (or dairy-free alternative)
- 1 cup fresh spinach
- 1 frozen banana
- ½ cup frozen blueberries
- 2 tablespoons pumpkin seeds
- 1 tablespoon ground flaxseed
- ½ cup cooled green tea (optional, for extra polyphenols)
- ½ cup ice

METHOD

1. Add all ingredients to a high-speed blender.
2. Blend on high for 60-90 seconds until completely smooth.
3. Add more liquid if too thick or ice if too thin.
4. Pour into glasses and serve at once.

THE SCIENCE Kefir has 30-40 probiotic strains (improves gut-brain communication). Magnesium from spinach and pumpkin seeds calms anxiety (Nutrients, 2019). Green tea's L-theanine reduces cortisol while enhancing focus. Flax provides omega-3 precursors.

NUTRITIONAL HIGHLIGHTS ~280 calories per serving | Rich in: Probiotics, Magnesium (120mg), Fiber (8g), Antioxidants

VARIATIONS

- Extra protein: Add protein powder or Greek yogurt
- Creamier: Add ½ avocado
- Different greens: Use kale or Swiss chard
- Berry swap: Try strawberries, raspberries, or mixed berries

STORAGE Best fresh. Can refrigerate up to 24 hours; shake well before drinking.

Recipe 4: Golden Turmeric Breakfast Bowl

Anti-inflammatory • Joint health • Cancer prevention

SERVES: 2 | **PREP:** 5 min | **COOK:** 10 min

WHY IT WORKS *Turmeric's curcumin reduces inflammation (lowers CRP and IL-6). Black pepper increases curcumin absorption by 2,000%. Quinoa provides complete protein. Perfect for those managing arthritis, chronic pain, or inflammatory conditions.*

INGREDIENTS

For the bowl:

- 1 cup quinoa, rinsed
- 1½ cups coconut milk (or almond milk)
- ½ cup water
- 1 teaspoon ground turmeric
- ½ teaspoon ground cinnamon
- ½ teaspoon ground ginger
- ¼ teaspoon black pepper (critical for curcumin absorption)
- Pinch of salt

Toppings:

- ½ cup fresh mango or pineapple, diced
- ¼ cup chopped almonds
- 2 tablespoons unsweetened coconut flakes
- 1 tablespoon chia seeds
- Optional: drizzle of honey

METHOD

1. In a medium saucepan, combine quinoa, coconut milk, water, turmeric, cinnamon, ginger, pepper, and salt.
2. Bring to a boil over medium-high heat.
3. Reduce heat to low, cover, and simmer for 15 minutes until quinoa is tender and liquid absorbed.
4. Remove from heat and let sit covered for 5 minutes.
5. Fluff with a fork and divide between two bowls.
6. Top with mango, almonds, coconut, and chia seeds.
7. Drizzle with honey if desired.

THE SCIENCE Curcumin reduces inflammatory markers (Journal of Medicinal Food, 2016). Black pepper's piperine increases bioavailability 2,000% (Planta Medica, 1998). Quinoa provides all 9 essential amino acids. Coconut provides MCTs for brain energy.

NUTRITIONAL HIGHLIGHTS ~420 calories per serving | Rich in: Protein (12g), Fiber (8g), Curcumin, Healthy fats

VARIATIONS

- Savory version: Skip sweet toppings, add avocado and hemp seeds
- Extra protein: Top with Greek yogurt
- Different spices: Add cardamom or nutmeg
- Seasonal fruit: Use berries, apple, or pear instead of mango

STORAGE Refrigerate base for up to 4 days. Reheat with splash of milk, add fresh toppings.

Recipe 5: Chia Pudding Three Ways

Omega-3s • Digestive health • Blood sugar stability

SERVES: 4 | **PREP:** 5 min + overnight | **COOK:** 0 min

WHY IT WORKS *Chia seeds provide 5g fiber and 2.5g omega-3s per table-spoon. They stabilize blood sugar, support gut health, and keep you full for hours. Perfect make-ahead breakfast that travels well.*

BASE INGREDIENTS

- ½ cup chia seeds
- 2 cups almond milk (or milk of choice)
- 1 teaspoon vanilla extract
- Pinch of salt
- Optional: 1-2 tablespoons maple syrup or honey

METHOD

1. In a large jar or bowl, whisk together milk, vanilla, salt, and sweetener if using.
2. Add chia seeds and whisk vigorously for 30 seconds to prevent clumping.
3. Let sit for 5 minutes, then whisk again.
4. Cover and refrigerate overnight (or minimum 4 hours).
5. Stir before serving and divide among 4 containers.

VARIATION 1: BERRY ANTIOXIDANT

Toppings:

- 1 cup mixed berries (blueberries, strawberries, raspberries)
- ¼ cup chopped walnuts
- Fresh mint

Benefits: Richest source of antioxidants for brain protection and anti-aging.

VARIATION 2: TROPICAL ENERGY

Toppings:

- ½ cup diced mango
- ½ cup diced pineapple
- 2 tablespoons unsweetened coconut flakes
- 2 tablespoons macadamia nuts, chopped

Benefits: Vitamin C for immune support, MCTs for brain energy

VARIATION 3: CHOCOLATE PROTEIN

Add to base:

- 2 tablespoons cocoa powder
- 2 tablespoons protein powder Toppings:
- Sliced banana
- 2 tablespoons almond butter
- Cacao nibs

Benefits: Higher protein for muscle recovery, polyphenols from cocoa

THE SCIENCE Chia seeds absorb 10x their weight in liquid, creating gel that slows glucose absorption. Omega-3s (ALA) support cardiovascular health. Fiber feeds beneficial gut bacteria.

NUTRITIONAL HIGHLIGHTS ~240 calories per serving (base) | Rich in: Fiber (10g), Omega-3s (2.5g), Calcium, Magnesium

STORAGE Prepare base up to 5 days ahead. Add toppings fresh each day.

Recipe 6: Flaxseed Banana Pancakes

Heart health • Digestive health • Cancer prevention

SERVES: 4 (makes 8 pancakes) | **PREP:** 10 min | **COOK:** 15 min

WHY IT WORKS *Flaxseed provides lignans (reduce breast cancer risk) and omega-3s. Bananas add potassium (blood pressure regulation) and natural sweetness. Whole grain flour provides sustained energy. Perfect weekend breakfast that feels indulgent but nourishes deeply.*

INGREDIENTS

Dry ingredients:

- 1 cup whole wheat flour (or oat flour for gluten-free)
- ¼ cup ground flaxseed
- 2 teaspoons baking powder
- 1 teaspoon cinnamon
- ¼ teaspoon salt Wet ingredients:
- 2 ripe bananas, mashed
- 1 cup almond milk (or milk of choice)
- 2 tablespoons maple syrup
- 1 teaspoon vanilla extract
- 2 tablespoons melted coconut oil

For cooking:

- Coconut oil or olive oil spray
- For serving:
- Fresh berries
- Chopped walnuts
- Pure maple syrup (optional)

METHOD

1. In a large bowl, whisk together flour, flaxseed, baking powder, cinnamon, and salt.
2. In another bowl, combine mashed bananas, milk, maple syrup, vanilla, and melted coconut oil.
3. Pour wet ingredients into dry and stir until just combined (do not over-mix; some lumps are okay).
4. Let batter rest for 5 minutes (flax absorbs liquid).
5. Heat a griddle or large skillet over medium heat. Lightly oil.
6. Pour ¼ cup batter per pancake onto hot griddle.
7. Cook until bubbles form on surface and edges look set (2-3 minutes).
8. Flip and cook another 2 minutes until golden brown.
9. Serve warm with berries, walnuts, and a light drizzle of maple syrup.

THE SCIENCE Flaxseed lignans modulate estrogen metabolism, reducing breast cancer risk (Breast Cancer Research, 2017). Omega-3s (ALA) support cardiovascular health. Whole grains provide sustained glucose release, preventing energy crashes.

NUTRITIONAL HIGHLIGHTS ~280 calories per serving (2 pancakes) | Rich in: Fiber (8g), Omega-3s (2g), Lignans, Potassium

VARIATIONS

- Blueberry: Fold ½ cup blueberries into batter
- Protein boost: Add protein powder to dry ingredients
- Gluten-free: Use certified GF oat flour
- Vegan: Already vegan as written

STORAGE Refrigerate cooked pancakes up to 3 days. Freeze up to 3 months (separate with parchment paper). Reheat in toaster or oven.

Recipe 7: Turmeric Lentil Soup

Anti-inflammatory • Heart health • Digestive support

SERVES: 6 | **PREP:** 15 min | **COOK:** 40 min

WHY IT WORKS *This Sardinian-inspired soup delivers soluble fiber (lowers cholesterol), plant protein (stabilizes blood sugar), and curcumin (calms systemic inflammation). Perfect for meal prep—it improves with time and freezes beautifully.*

INGREDIENTS

Base:

- 3 tablespoons extra virgin olive oil
- 1 large onion, chopped
- 2 carrots, diced
- 2 celery stalks, diced
- 4 garlic cloves, minced

Soup:

- 1 cup brown or green lentils, rinsed
- 1 can (14 oz) crushed tomatoes
- 6 cups vegetable broth or water
- 2 teaspoons ground turmeric
- 1 teaspoon ground cumin
- ½ teaspoon black pepper (activates curcumin)
- 1 teaspoon salt

Finish:

- 2 cups chopped spinach or kale
- Juice of 1 lemon
- Extra olive oil for drizzling
- Fresh parsley for garnish

METHOD

1. Heat olive oil in a large pot over medium heat.
2. Add onion, carrots, and celery. Sauté until softened (6-8 minutes).
3. Add garlic, turmeric, cumin, and black pepper. Stir for 1 minute until fragrant.
4. Add tomatoes, lentils, broth, and salt. Bring to a boil.
5. Reduce heat and simmer uncovered for 30-40 minutes until lentils are tender.
6. Stir in greens during the last 2 minutes until wilted.
7. Remove from heat, add lemon juice.
8. Serve in bowls with a drizzle of olive oil and fresh parsley.

THE SCIENCE Lentils' soluble fiber lowers LDL cholesterol 5-10% (The Lancet, 2019). Turmeric's curcumin reduces CRP and IL-6 inflammatory markers (American Journal of Clinical Nutrition, 2016). Black pepper increases curcumin absorption 2,000%.

NUTRITIONAL HIGHLIGHTS ~250 calories per serving | Rich in: Fiber (12g), Protein (11g), Iron, Folate, Curcumin

VARIATIONS

- Creamier: Blend 1 cup of soup and stir back in
- Extra protein: Add quinoa in last 15 minutes
- Mediterranean: Top with feta and fresh oregano
- Spicier: Add cayenne or red pepper flakes

STORAGE Refrigerate up to 5 days. Freezes beautifully for 3 months. Reheat gently, add water if needed to thin.

Recipe 8: Mediterranean Grain Bowl

Prevention • Heart health • Weight management

SERVES: 4 | **PREP:** 15 min (if grains pre-cooked) | **COOK:** 0 min

WHY IT WORKS *This bowl mirrors Blue Zones eating patterns: complete protein from grain-legume pairing, resistant starch (feeds gut bacteria), polyphenols from olive oil, steady energy without crashes. The exact combination associated with reduced cardiovascular and cancer risk.*

INGREDIENTS

Base:

- 2 cups cooked quinoa or barley (cooled)
- 1 can (15 oz) chickpeas, drained and rinsed

Vegetables:

- 1 cucumber, diced
- 1 cup cherry tomatoes, halved
- ½ red onion, thinly sliced
- ½ cup Kalamata olives, pitted

Dressing:

- 4 tablespoons extra virgin olive oil
- Juice of 1 lemon
- 1 teaspoon dried oregano
- 1 garlic clove, minced
- Salt and pepper to taste

Toppings:

- ¼ cup chopped fresh parsley
- ¼ cup chopped fresh mint
- ¼ cup crumbled feta (optional)
- ¼ cup chopped walnuts

METHOD

1. In a large bowl, combine quinoa and chickpeas.
2. Add cucumber, tomatoes, onion, and olives.
3. In a small bowl, whisk together olive oil, lemon juice, oregano, garlic, salt, and pepper.
4. Pour dressing over grain mixture and toss gently.
5. Fold in fresh herbs.
6. Top with feta if using, and walnuts.
7. Serve at room temperature or chilled.

THE SCIENCE Chickpeas provide resistant starch that lowers glucose (Diabetes Care, 2018). Quinoa supplies all 9 essential amino acids. Tomatoes bring lycopene (reduces prostate cancer risk, Cancer Epidemiology, 2016). Olive oil polyphenols improve endothelial function.

NUTRITIONAL HIGHLIGHTS ~420 calories per serving | Rich in: Fiber (11g), Protein (14g), Polyphenols, Complete amino acids

VARIATIONS

- Winter: Swap fresh vegetables for roasted ones
- Extra satiety: Add sliced avocado
- More protein: Top with grilled chicken, tofu, or salmon
- Different grains: Use brown rice, farro, or bulgur

STORAGE Components can be prepped ahead. Dress just before serving for best texture. Lasts 4 days refrigerated.

Recipe 9: Sardinian Minestrone

Longevity • Heart health • Digestive support

SERVES: 8 | **PREP:** 15 min | **COOK:** 50 min

WHY IT WORKS *This soup appears in the lives of Sardinian centenarians because it is inexpensive, nourishing, and deeply satisfying. Legume-grain pairing provides broader amino acid profile, fiber supports cholesterol reduction, rosemary adds antioxidants.*

INGREDIENTS

Base:

- 3 tablespoons extra virgin olive oil
- 1 onion, diced
- 2 carrots, diced
- 2 celery stalks, diced
- 4 garlic cloves, minced

Soup:

- 1 can (15 oz) white beans or mixed beans
- ½ cup pearl barley
- 1 can (14 oz) diced tomatoes
- 6 cups vegetable broth or water
- 2 cups chopped cabbage or kale
- 1 zucchini, diced (optional)
- 2 teaspoons dried rosemary
- 1 teaspoon dried thyme
- 2 bay leaves
- Salt and pepper to taste

Finish:

- Extra olive oil for drizzling
- Fresh parsley
- Optional: spoonful of pesto per bowl

METHOD

1. Heat olive oil in a large pot over medium heat.
2. Sauté onion, carrots, and celery until softened (6-8 minutes).
3. Add garlic and cook for 1 minute.
4. Add beans, barley, tomatoes, broth, rosemary, thyme, and bay leaves.
5. Bring to a boil, then reduce heat and simmer for 40 minutes.
6. Add cabbage or kale and zucchini if using. Simmer for 10 more minutes.
7. Remove bay leaves. Season with salt and pepper.
8. Serve in bowls with a drizzle of olive oil and fresh parsley.
9. Optional: Stir in a spoonful of pesto at the table.

THE SCIENCE Barley lowers cholesterol and improves gut microbiota (Nutrients, 2018). Beans supply folate and resistant starch. Cruciferous greens activate detoxification enzymes that reduce cancer risk. Rosemary provides rosmarinic acid (antioxidant, anti-inflammatory).

NUTRITIONAL HIGHLIGHTS ~220 calories per serving | Rich in: Fiber (9g), Protein (8g), Iron, Folate

VARIATIONS

- Extra vegetables: Add green beans, spinach, or Swiss chard
- Creamier: Mash some beans against the side of the pot
- Heartier: Add whole grain pasta in the last 10 minutes
- Pesto: Adds healthy fats and intense flavor

STORAGE Refrigerates beautifully for 5 days. Freezes for 3 months. Flavors deepen overnight.

Recipe 10: Chickpea "Tuna" Salad Wrap

Plant-based protein • Quick lunch • Heart health

SERVES: 4 | **PREP:** 10 min | **COOK:** 0 min

WHY IT WORKS *Chickpeas provide plant protein and resistant starch (gut health). Nori adds iodine and umami "fish" flavor. Avocado supplies healthy fats. Perfect for meal prep—make the filling ahead and assemble wraps fresh.*

INGREDIENTS

For the filling:

- 2 cans (15 oz each) chickpeas, drained and rinsed
- 1 avocado, mashed
- 2 tablespoons tahini
- 2 tablespoons lemon juice
- 1 tablespoon Dijon mustard
- 1 nori sheet, crumbled (for "fishy" flavor)
- ¼ cup diced celery
- ¼ cup diced red onion
- 2 tablespoons fresh dill or parsley, chopped
- Salt and pepper to taste

For assembly:

- 4 whole grain wraps or large lettuce leaves
- 2 cups mixed greens
- 1 tomato, sliced
- ½ cucumber, thinly sliced

METHOD

1. In a large bowl, mash chickpeas with a fork or potato masher until mostly broken down but still chunky.
2. Add mashed avocado, tahini, lemon juice, mustard, and crumbled nori. Mix well.
3. Fold in celery, onion, and fresh herbs. Season with salt and pepper.
4. Taste and adjust seasoning.
5. To assemble wraps: lay out wrap, add greens, spoon chickpea mixture down the center, top with tomato and cucumber.
6. Roll tightly, tucking in sides as you go.
7. Cut in half diagonally.

THE SCIENCE Chickpeas provide resistant starch that feeds beneficial gut bacteria and lowers glucose. Tahini adds calcium and sesame lignans. Avocado provides monounsaturated fats (heart protection). Nori contributes iodine for thyroid function.

NUTRITIONAL HIGHLIGHTS ~380 calories per serving | Rich in: Fiber (12g), Protein (13g), Healthy fats, Iodine

VARIATIONS

- Crunchy: Add diced apple or grapes
- Spicy: Add sriracha or cayenne
- Omega-3 boost: Add ground flaxseed or hemp seeds
- Low carb: Use large lettuce leaves instead of wraps

STORAGE Refrigerate filling up to 4 days. Assemble wraps fresh for best texture, or prep and wrap tightly in parchment for grab-and-go.

Recipe 11: Anti-Inflammatory Golden Lentils

Arthritis • Chronic pain • Depression

SERVES: 6 | **PREP:** 10 min | **COOK:** 35 min

WHY IT WORKS *This dish combines cholesterol-lowering lentils with turmeric's anti-inflammatory curcumin. Perfect for managing arthritis, heart disease, depression, or chronic inflammation. Comfort food that heals.*

INGREDIENTS

Base:

- 2 tablespoons coconut oil or olive oil
- 1 onion, diced
- 3 garlic cloves, minced
- 1 tablespoon fresh ginger, grated

Lentils:

- 1 cup red lentils, rinsed
- 1 can (14 oz) coconut milk
- 2 cups vegetable broth
- 2 teaspoons ground turmeric
- 1 teaspoon ground cumin
- ½ teaspoon black pepper (activates curcumin)
- 1 teaspoon salt

Finish:

- 2 cups fresh spinach
- Juice of 1 lime
- Fresh cilantro, chopped

METHOD

1. Heat oil in a large pot over medium heat.
2. Sauté onion until softened (5 minutes).
3. Add garlic and ginger, stir for 1 minute until fragrant.
4. Add turmeric, cumin, and black pepper. Stir for 30 seconds.
5. Add lentils, coconut milk, and broth. Bring to a boil.
6. Reduce heat and simmer for 20-25 minutes until lentils are soft.
7. Stir in spinach until wilted.
8. Remove from heat, add lime juice.
9. Serve over brown rice or quinoa, garnished with fresh cilantro.

THE SCIENCE Turmeric's curcumin reduces inflammatory markers like CRP and IL-6 (Journal of Medicinal Food, 2016). Black pepper increases curcumin absorption 2,000%. Lentils stabilize blood sugar and lower cholesterol. Coconut milk adds MCTs for brain support.

NUTRITIONAL HIGHLIGHTS ~280 calories per serving | Rich in: Fiber (8g), Protein (10g), Curcumin, Iron

VARIATIONS

- Extra vegetables: Add sweet potato or carrots
- Spicier: Add cayenne or red chili flakes
- Depression support: Serve with salmon on the side (omega-3 boost)
- Creamier: Use full-fat coconut milk

STORAGE Refrigerate up to 5 days. Freezes well for 3 months. Reheat gently, add liquid if needed.

Recipe 12: Quick Black Bean Buddha Bowl

Blood sugar stability • Plant protein • Heart health

SERVES: 2 | **PREP:** 10 min | **COOK:** 5 min

WHY IT WORKS *Black beans stabilize blood sugar and provide magnesium. Avocado adds potassium (lowers blood pressure). Quick-pickled vegetables add probiotics. Perfect for busy weekdays—nutrient-dense and ready in 15 minutes.*

INGREDIENTS

Base:

- 1 cup cooked brown rice or quinoa

Bowl components:

- 1 can (15 oz) black beans, drained and rinsed
- 1 avocado, sliced
- 1 cup cherry tomatoes, halved
- 1 cup corn (fresh, frozen, or canned)
- 2 cups mixed greens or shredded cabbage

Quick-pickled onions:

- ½ red onion, thinly sliced
- ¼ cup lime juice
- Pinch of salt

Dressing:

- 2 tablespoons tahini
- 2 tablespoons lime juice
- 2 tablespoons water
- 1 garlic clove, minced
- Salt and pepper

METHOD

1. Make quick-pickled onions: combine sliced onion, lime juice, and salt in a small bowl. Let sit while you prepare the rest.
2. Warm black beans gently in a small pot with a splash of water and cumin if desired.
3. Make dressing: whisk together tahini, lime juice, water, garlic, salt, and pepper until smooth.
4. Assemble bowls: divide rice between two bowls. Top each with black beans, avocado, tomatoes, corn, and greens.
5. Add quick-pickled onions.
6. Drizzle with tahini dressing.

THE SCIENCE Black beans provide resistant starch and magnesium (calms nervous system). Avocado adds potassium (lowers blood pressure 4-5 mmHg, Hypertension, 2019). Fermented onions contribute probiotics for gut health.

NUTRITIONAL HIGHLIGHTS ~480 calories per serving | Rich in: Fiber (16g), Protein (15g), Magnesium, Potassium

VARIATIONS

- Add protein: Top with grilled chicken, tofu, or tempeh
- Spicy: Add jalapeños or spicy sauce
- Different grains: Use farro, bulgur, or cauliflower rice
- Extra crunch: Add pepitas or sunflower seeds

STORAGE Prep components separately. Assemble fresh for best texture. Components last 3-4 days refrigerated.

Recipe 13: Pomegranate Salmon

Heart health • Cancer prevention • Brain function

SERVES: 4 | **PREP:** 10 min | **COOK:** 15 min

WHY IT WORKS *This dish unites anti-inflammatory omega-3s (salmon) with powerful antioxidants (pomegranate). Cancer survivors and heart patients receive help from this combination—it feels like celebration food but functions as therapy.*

INGREDIENTS

For the salmon:

- 4 salmon fillets (4-6 oz each)
- 2 tablespoons extra virgin olive oil
- Salt and pepper
- 1 lemon, sliced

For serving:

- 4 cups fresh spinach
- 1 cup pomegranate arils (seeds)
- ¼ cup fresh parsley, chopped
- 2 tablespoons olive oil
- Juice of ½ lemon

METHOD

1. Preheat oven to 375°F (190°C).
2. Line a baking sheet with parchment paper.
3. Rub salmon fillets with 1 tablespoon olive oil, season with salt and pepper.
4. Place lemon slices on top of each fillet.
5. Bake for 12-15 minutes until salmon flakes easily with a fork (do not overcook).
6. While salmon bakes, heat remaining olive oil in a large skillet over medium heat.
7. Add spinach and sauté until just wilted (2 minutes). Add lemon juice.
8. Divide spinach among four plates.
9. Top with salmon fillet, scatter pomegranate seeds, finish with fresh parsley.

THE SCIENCE Salmon provides DHA omega-3s (reduce arrhythmia, stabilize mood, JAMA, 2012). Pomegranate arils are rich in punicalagins (reduce arterial plaque, Atherosclerosis, 2015). Spinach supplies iron and folate for red blood cell health.

NUTRITIONAL HIGHLIGHTS ~380 calories per serving | Rich in: Omega-3s (2g), Protein (32g), Vitamin K, Iron, Polyphenols

VARIATIONS

- Budget: Use sardines on whole grain toast with pomegranate
- Spiced: Add cumin and coriander to spinach
- Make ahead: Cook salmon, refrigerate, serve cold over salad

STORAGE Refrigerate cooked salmon up to 3 days. Best fresh, but left-overs work beautifully in salads.

Recipe 14: One-Pan Mediterranean Chicken

Easy weeknight • Heart health • Family-friendly

SERVES: 4 | **PREP:** 15 min | **COOK:** 40 min

WHY IT WORKS *Sheet pan dinners minimize cleanup while maximizing nutrition. Chicken provides lean protein, vegetables deliver antioxidants, olive oil and lemon create Mediterranean magic. Perfect for busy families.*

INGREDIENTS

For the chicken:

- 4 chicken thighs or breasts (bone-in, skin-on for more flavor)
- 2 tablespoons extra virgin olive oil
- 2 teaspoons dried oregano
- 1 teaspoon paprika
- Salt and pepper

For the vegetables:

- 1 lb baby potatoes, halved
- 1 red bell pepper, cut into chunks
- 1 yellow bell pepper, cut into chunks
- 1 red onion, cut into wedges
- 1 cup cherry tomatoes
- 1 cup Kalamata olives
- 4 garlic cloves, smashed
- 2 tablespoons olive oil
- Fresh lemon wedges
- Fresh oregano or parsley for garnish

METHOD

1. Preheat oven to 425°F (220°C).
2. In a small bowl, mix 2 tablespoons olive oil with oregano, paprika, salt, and pepper.
3. Rub mixture all over chicken pieces.
4. On a large sheet pan, toss potatoes, peppers, onion, tomatoes, olives, and garlic with remaining olive oil, salt, and pepper.
5. Nestle chicken pieces among vegetables.
6. Roast for 35-40 minutes until chicken reaches 165°F internal temperature and vegetables are tender and caramelized.
7. Squeeze fresh lemon over everything before serving.
8. Garnish with fresh herbs.

THE SCIENCE Chicken provides lean protein without saturated fat overload. Bell peppers deliver vitamin C (immune support). Tomatoes provide lycopene (cardiovascular protection). Olive oil and oregano add polyphenols. Olives contribute healthy monounsaturated fats.

NUTRITIONAL HIGHLIGHTS ~420 calories per serving | Rich in: Protein (32g), Vitamin C, Lycopene, Healthy fats

VARIATIONS

- Different vegetables: Use Brussels sprouts, zucchini, or carrots
- Spicy: Add red pepper flakes
- Greek-style: Add crumbled feta after roasting
- Meal **PREP:** Makes excellent leftovers for lunch bowls

STORAGE Refrigerate up to 4 days. Reheat in oven to support crispy skin or enjoy cold in salads.

Recipe 15: Lentil Bolognese

Plant-based comfort • Heart health • Budget-friendly

SERVES: 6 | **PREP:** 15 min | **COOK:** 35 min

WHY IT WORKS *This plant-based take on classic Bolognese delivers the comfort of pasta night with the nutrition of lentils. Fiber lowers cholesterol, plant protein stabilizes blood sugar, and the familiar flavors make healthy eating feel indulgent.*

INGREDIENTS

For the sauce:

- 2 tablespoons extra virgin olive oil
- 1 onion, finely diced
- 2 carrots, finely diced
- 2 celery stalks, finely diced
- 4 garlic cloves, minced
- 1 cup brown or green lentils, rinsed
- 1 can (28 oz) crushed tomatoes
- 1 can (6 oz) tomato paste
- 2 cups vegetable broth
- 2 teaspoons dried oregano
- 1 teaspoon dried basil
- ½ teaspoon red pepper flakes (optional)
- 2 bay leaves
- Salt and pepper to taste

For serving:

- 1 lb whole grain pasta
- Fresh basil for garnish
- Nutritional yeast or Parmesan (optional)

METHOD

1. Heat olive oil in a large pot over medium heat.
2. Add onion, carrots, and celery (traditional "soffritto"). Sauté until softened (8-10 minutes).
3. Add garlic and cook for 1 minute.
4. Add lentils, crushed tomatoes, tomato paste, broth, oregano, basil, red pepper flakes, and bay leaves.
5. Bring to a boil, then reduce heat and simmer uncovered for 30-35 minutes until lentils are tender and sauce has thickened.
6. Remove bay leaves. Season with salt and pepper.
7. Meanwhile, cook pasta according to package directions. Reserve 1 cup pasta water before draining.
8. Toss pasta with sauce, adding reserved pasta water if needed to reach desired consistency.
9. Serve with fresh basil and nutritional yeast or Parmesan.

THE SCIENCE Lentils provide soluble fiber (lowers LDL cholesterol). Plant protein stabilizes blood sugar without saturated fat. Tomatoes deliver lycopene (prostate health). Carrots and celery add carotenoids and flavonoids.

NUTRITIONAL HIGHLIGHTS ~420 calories per serving | Rich in: Fiber (14g), Protein (16g), Iron, Lycopene

VARIATIONS

- Extra vegetables: Add mushrooms, zucchini, or spinach
- Gluten-free: Use chickpea or lentil pasta
- Creamier: Stir in cashew cream or coconut milk
- Meal **PREP:** Sauce freezes beautifully for 3 months

STORAGE Refrigerate sauce up to 5 days. Freeze up to 3 months. Cook pasta fresh when ready to serve.

Recipe 16: Miso-Glazed Cod with Ginger Bok Choy

Brain health • Anti-aging • Asian-inspired

SERVES: 4 | **PREP:** 10 min + 30 min marinating | **COOK:** 15 min

WHY IT WORKS *Cod provides lean protein and omega-3s. Miso delivers probiotics and umami depth. Ginger is anti-inflammatory. Bok choy supplies calcium and vitamin K. Elegant enough for guests, simple enough for weeknights.*

INGREDIENTS

For the miso glaze:

- 3 tablespoons white miso paste
- 2 tablespoons mirin (or rice vinegar + 1 tsp honey)
- 1 tablespoon low-sodium soy sauce or tamari
- 1 tablespoon sesame oil
- 1 tablespoon fresh ginger, grated
- 2 garlic cloves, minced

For the fish:

- 4 cod fillets (6 oz each)

For the bok choy:

- 1 tablespoon sesame oil
- 4 heads baby bok choy, halved lengthwise
- 2 garlic cloves, minced
- 1 tablespoon fresh ginger, grated
- 2 tablespoons water
- 1 tablespoon sesame seeds
- Sliced green onions for garnish

METHOD

1. Make miso glaze: whisk together miso, mirin, soy sauce, sesame oil, ginger, and garlic.
2. Place cod fillets in a shallow dish. Pour half the glaze over fish, turning to coat. Marinate 30 minutes (or up to 2 hours) in refrigerator.
3. Preheat oven to 400°F (200°C).
4. Line a baking sheet with parchment. Place marinated cod on sheet.
5. Bake for 12-15 minutes until fish flakes easily.
6. Meanwhile, heat sesame oil in a large skillet over medium-high heat.
7. Add bok choy cut side down. Cook without moving for 2-3 minutes until browned.
8. Flip, add garlic, ginger, and water. Cover and steam for 2 minutes until tender.
9. Serve cod over bok choy, drizzle with reserved glaze, sprinkle with sesame seeds and green onions.

THE SCIENCE Cod provides lean protein and omega-3s. Miso has probiotics (gut-brain health). Ginger reduces inflammation and nausea. Bok choy is high in calcium and vitamin K (bone health). Sesame provides lignans and healthy fats.

NUTRITIONAL HIGHLIGHTS ~280 calories per serving | Rich in: Protein (34g), Probiotics, Calcium, Omega-3s

VARIATIONS

- Different fish: Use halibut, salmon, or tofu
- Spicier: Add sriracha to glaze
- Grain base: Serve over brown rice or quinoa
- Extra vegetables: Add shiitake mushrooms or snap peas

STORAGE Best fresh. Cod can be refrigerated up to 2 days. Reheat gently to avoid overcooking.

Recipe 17: Stuffed Bell Peppers with Quinoa and Black Beans

Complete protein • Colorful • Crowd-pleaser

SERVES: 4 | **PREP:** 20 min | **COOK:** 35 min

WHY IT WORKS *Bell peppers provide vitamin C (immune support). Quinoa-bean combination delivers complete protein. Tomatoes add lycopene. Cumin and chili powder bring anti-inflammatory compounds. Beautiful presentation makes healthy eating exciting.*

INGREDIENTS

For the peppers:

- 4 large bell peppers (any color), tops cut off, seeds removed

For the filling:

- 1 tablespoon olive oil
- 1 onion, diced
- 3 garlic cloves, minced
- 1 can (15 oz) black beans, drained
- 1½ cups cooked quinoa
- 1 can (14 oz) diced tomatoes, drained
- 1 cup corn (fresh, frozen, or canned)
- 1 teaspoon ground cumin
- 1 teaspoon chili powder
- ½ teaspoon smoked paprika
- Salt and pepper
- ½ cup shredded cheese (optional)
- Fresh cilantro for garnish

METHOD

1. Preheat oven to 375°F (190°C).
2. Bring a large pot of water to boil. Add bell peppers and blanch for 3 minutes. Drain and set aside.
3. Heat olive oil in a large skillet. Sauté onion until softened (5 minutes).
4. Add garlic and cook for 1 minute.
5. Add black beans, quinoa, tomatoes, corn, cumin, chili powder, paprika, salt, and pepper. Stir to combine and heat through.
6. Place blanched peppers in a baking dish, standing upright.
7. Fill each pepper with quinoa mixture, packing gently.
8. Top with cheese if using.
9. Cover with foil and bake for 25 minutes.
10. Remove foil and bake 5 more minutes until cheese melts.
11. Garnish with fresh cilantro.

THE SCIENCE Bell peppers provide vitamin C (one pepper = 169% daily value). Quinoa-bean pairing creates complete protein with all 9 essential amino acids. Cumin and chili powder have capsaicin and curcuminoids (anti-inflammatory).

NUTRITIONAL HIGHLIGHTS ~340 calories per serving | Rich in: Fiber (12g), Protein (13g), Vitamin C (200% DV), Complete amino acids

VARIATIONS

- Different grains: Use brown rice, bulgur, or cauliflower rice
- Extra vegetables: Add diced zucchini or mushrooms to filling
- Vegan: Skip cheese, top with nutritional yeast
- Spicier: Add jalapeños or cayenne

STORAGE Refrigerate up to 4 days. Reheat in oven or microwave. Freezes well (wrap individually) for 3 months.

Recipe 18: Sheet Pan Roasted Vegetable Medley

Versatile • Batch-cooking • Anti-inflammatory

SERVES: 6 | **PREP:** 15 min | **COOK:** 30 min

WHY IT WORKS *Roasting concentrates flavor and preserves antioxi-dants. Olive oil increases absorption of carotenoids and polyphenols. These vegetables provide a spectrum of vitamins and phytochemicals. Perfect batch-cooking strategy—make once, eat all week.*

INGREDIENTS

Choose 8-10 cups total of:

- 2 cups carrots, cut into sticks
- 2 zucchinis, chopped
- 1 red bell pepper, sliced
- 1 yellow bell pepper, sliced
- 1 red onion, cut into wedges
- 1 small eggplant, cubed
- 2 cups broccoli florets
- 2 cups Brussels sprouts, halved

For roasting:

- ¼ cup extra virgin olive oil
- 1 teaspoon salt
- ½ teaspoon black pepper
- 1 tablespoon fresh rosemary (or 1 teaspoon dried)
- 1 tablespoon fresh thyme (or 1 teaspoon dried)

To finish:

- Juice of 1 lemon
- Extra drizzle of olive oil

METHOD

1. Preheat oven to 425°F (220°C).
2. Cut all vegetables into similar-sized pieces for even roasting.
3. In a large bowl, toss vegetables with olive oil, salt, pepper, rosemary, and thyme until well coated.
4. Spread in a single layer on two large baking sheets (do not over-crowd—they will steam instead of roast).
5. Roast for 25-30 minutes, stirring halfway through, until edges are caramelized and vegetables are tender.
6. Remove from oven, squeeze lemon juice over top, drizzle with extra olive oil.

THE SCIENCE Roasting at high heat preserves antioxidants while enhancing flavor through caramelization. Olive oil increases absorption of carotenoids (beta-carotene, lycopene) by up to 400% (American Journal of Clinical Nutrition, 2004). These vegetables provide fiber, vitamin C, folate, and polyphenols.

NUTRITIONAL HIGHLIGHTS ~150 calories per serving | Rich in: Fiber (6g), Vitamin C, Carotenoids, Polyphenols

VARIATIONS

- Complete meal: Toss with cooked chickpeas and serve with whole grain bread
- Mediterranean: Add olives and feta after roasting
- Spicy: Sprinkle with red pepper flakes before roasting
- Asian-inspired: Use sesame oil, add ginger and garlic

STORAGE Refrigerate up to 5 days. Reheat in oven or eat cold in salads or wraps. Perfect for meal prep.

PART D: SNACKS & SIDES

Recipe 19: Roasted Chickpeas Three Ways

Crunchy • Protein • Portable

SERVES: 4 | **PREP:** 5 min | **COOK:** 30 min

WHY IT WORKS *Chickpeas provide plant protein and resistant starch. Roasting creates satisfying crunch without deep-frying. Perfect replacement for chips—nutrient-dense, portable, and addictive in the best way.*

BASE RECIPE

Ingredients:

- 2 cans (15 oz each) chickpeas, drained and rinsed
- 2 tablespoons extra virgin olive oil
- Salt to taste

Method:

1. Preheat oven to 400°F (200°C).
2. Pat chickpeas very dry with paper towels (critical for crispiness).
3. Toss with olive oil and salt.
4. Spread on a baking sheet in single layer.
5. Roast for 25-30 minutes, shaking pan every 10 minutes, until golden and crispy.
6. Let cool completely (they crisp up more as they cool).

VARIATION 1: SAVORY GARLIC HERB

Add before roasting:

- 1 teaspoon garlic powder
- 1 teaspoon dried rosemary
- ½ teaspoon black pepper

Benefits: Heart health, anti-inflammatory

VARIATION 2: SMOKY CHILI LIME

Add before roasting:

- 1 teaspoon chili powder
- 1 teaspoon smoked paprika
- ½ teaspoon cumin
- Juice of 1 lime (add after roasting)

Benefits: Metabolism boost, vitamin C

VARIATION 3: CINNAMON MAPLE (SWEET)

Add before roasting:

- 1 teaspoon cinnamon
- 2 tablespoons maple syrup
- Pinch of sea salt

Method notes: Roast at 375°F to prevent maple from burning

Benefits: Satisfies sweet tooth with fiber and protein

THE SCIENCE Chickpeas provide resistant starch (feeds gut bacteria, lowers glucose). Plant protein keeps you full. Roasting (vs. frying) preserves nutrients without adding unhealthy fats.

NUTRITIONAL HIGHLIGHTS ~180 calories per serving | Rich in: Fiber (8g), Protein (8g), Iron

STORAGE Store in airtight container at room temperature up to 5 days. Recrisp in 300°F oven for 5 minutes if needed.

Recipe 20: Creamy Hummus

Protein • Prebiotic fiber • Versatile

SERVES: 8 (makes ~2 cups) | **PREP:** 10 min | **COOK:** 0 min

WHY IT WORKS *Chickpeas and tahini create complete protein. Garlic is prebiotic (feeds gut bacteria). Lemon adds vitamin C. Olive oil provides polyphenols. Perfect for snacking with vegetables or as sandwich spread.*

INGREDIENTS

- 2 cans (15 oz each) chickpeas, drained (reserve ¼ cup liquid)
- ⅓ cup tahini (sesame seed paste)
- ¼ cup extra virgin olive oil, plus more for drizzling
- 3 tablespoons lemon juice
- 2 garlic cloves
- 1 teaspoon ground cumin
- ½ teaspoon salt
- 2-4 tablespoons water or reserved chickpea liquid
- Paprika for garnish
- Fresh parsley for garnish

METHOD

1. In a food processor, combine chickpeas, tahini, olive oil, lemon juice, garlic, cumin, and salt.
2. Process for 1 minute, scraping down sides.
3. With motor running, slowly add water or chickpea liquid until desired consistency is reached (smooth and creamy).
4. Taste and adjust seasoning (more lemon, salt, or garlic as desired).
5. Transfer to a serving bowl.
6. Create a well in the center with the back of a spoon.
7. Drizzle with olive oil, sprinkle with paprika and parsley.

THE SCIENCE Chickpeas and tahini together provide complete protein. Garlic has inulin (prebiotic fiber that feeds beneficial bacteria). Tahini adds calcium and sesame lignans. Olive oil polyphenols reduce inflammation.

NUTRITIONAL HIGHLIGHTS ~140 calories per ¼ cup | Rich in: Protein (5g), Fiber (4g), Calcium, Iron

VARIATIONS

- Roasted red pepper: Blend in 1 roasted red pepper
- Spicy: Add cayenne or jalapeño
- Herb: Blend in fresh cilantro or parsley
- Beet: Blend in 1 cooked beet for beautiful pink color

STORAGE Refrigerate up to 7 days. Bring to room temperature before serving. Drizzle with fresh olive oil.

Recipe 21: Energy Balls

Pre-workout • Portable • Natural sweetness

SERVES: 12 balls | **PREP:** 15 min | **COOK:** 0 min

WHY IT WORKS *Dates provide natural sweetness and quick energy. Nuts add healthy fats and protein. Seeds deliver omega-3s and minerals. Perfect preworkout snack or healthy dessert—satisfies sweet tooth with nutrition.*

INGREDIENTS

Base:

- 1 cup Medjool dates, pitted (about 12 dates)
- 1 cup raw almonds or walnuts
- 2 tablespoons ground flaxseed
- 2 tablespoons chia seeds
- 2 tablespoons cocoa powder
- 1 teaspoon vanilla extract
- Pinch of salt

Optional mix-ins:

- 2 tablespoons mini dark chocolate chips
- 2 tablespoons unsweetened coconut flakes
- 1 tablespoon hemp seeds

For rolling:

- Cocoa powder, coconut flakes, or sesame seeds

METHOD

1. In a food processor, pulse nuts until finely chopped (do not over-process into butter).
2. Add dates, flaxseed, chia seeds, cocoa powder, vanilla, and salt.
3. Process until mixture comes together and forms a sticky dough (30-60 seconds).
4. If too dry, add water 1 teaspoon at a time. If too wet, add more nuts or cocoa powder.
5. Stir in optional mixins by hand.
6. Roll into 12 balls (about 1 tablespoon each).
7. Roll in cocoa powder, coconut, or sesame seeds if desired.
8. Refrigerate for 30 minutes to firm up.

THE SCIENCE Dates provide quick-digesting natural sugars for energy without refined sugar crash. Nuts and seeds add healthy fats and protein for sustained energy. Cocoa provides flavonoids (cardiovascular health). Flax and chia add omega-3s.

NUTRITIONAL HIGHLIGHTS ~120 calories per ball | Rich in: Fiber (3g), Healthy fats, Iron, Magnesium

VARIATIONS

- Peanut butter: Add 2 tablespoons natural peanut butter
- Matcha: Add 1 tablespoon matcha powder
- Protein boost: Add protein powder
- Different nuts: Try cashews, pecans, or sunflower seeds

STORAGE Refrigerate up to 2 weeks in airtight container. Freeze up to 3 months.

Recipe 22: Kale Chips

Crunchy • Low-calorie • Nutrient-dense

SERVES: 4 | **PREP:** 10 min | **COOK:** 20 min

WHY IT WORKS *Kale is a nutritional powerhouse (vitamin K, vitamin C, calcium). Baking creates chip-like crunch with minimal oil. Perfect replacement for potato chips—satisfies crunch craving with nutrition.*

INGREDIENTS

- 1 large bunch kale (about 8 cups loosely packed)
- 1-2 tablespoons extra virgin olive oil
- Sea salt to taste

Flavor options:

- Classic: Just salt
- Cheesy: 2 tablespoons nutritional yeast
- Spicy: ½ teaspoon cayenne or chili powder
- Garlic: 1 teaspoon garlic powder

METHOD

1. Preheat oven to 300°F (150°C) - low temperature prevents burning.
2. Wash kale and dry VERY thoroughly (moisture = soggy chips).
3. Remove thick stems and tear leaves into bite-sized pieces.
4. In a large bowl, massage kale with olive oil until every piece is lightly coated.
5. Add salt and any flavorings, toss to distribute.
6. Spread in a single layer on two baking sheets (do not overlap).
7. Bake for 15-20 minutes, rotating pans halfway through, until edges are crispy but not brown.
8. Let cool on pan for 5 minutes (they crisp up more as they cool).

THE SCIENCE Kale provides vitamin K (importantforbonehealthandbloodclotting), vitamin C (immune support), calcium (dairy-free source), and sulforaphane (cancerprotective compound). Low-temperature baking preserves nutrients.

NUTRITIONAL HIGHLIGHTS ~60 calories per serving | Rich in: Vitamin K (680% DV), Vitamin C (134% DV), Calcium

VARIATIONS

- Ranch: Nutritional yeast + garlic powder + onion powder
- BBQ: Smoked paprika + garlic powder + touch of maple syrup
- Sesame: Sesame oil instead of olive oil, sesame seeds

STORAGE Best eaten at once. Store in air-tight container at room temperature up to 2 days. Recrisp in 300°F oven for 3-5 minutes if needed.

Recipe 23: Golden Anti-Inflammatory Latte

Joint health • Digestion • Warming

SERVES: 2 | **PREP:** 5 min | **COOK:** 5 min

WHY IT WORKS *Turmeric's curcumin reduces inflammation (arthritis, chronic pain). Black pepper increases absorption. Ginger aids digestion and adds warmth. Perfect evening ritual or post-workout recovery.*

INGREDIENTS

- 2 cups unsweetened almond milk (or milk of choice)
- 1 teaspoon ground turmeric
- ½ teaspoon ground ginger
- ¼ teaspoon ground cinnamon
- Pinch of black pepper (critical for curcumin absorption)
- 1 teaspoon coconut oil or ghee
- 1-2 teaspoons honey or maple syrup (optional)
- Pinch of cardamom (optional)

METHOD

1. In a small saucepan, warm milk over medium heat (do not boil).
2. Whisk in turmeric, ginger, cinnamon, and black pepper.
3. Add coconut oil and whisk until melted and frothy.
4. Simmer gently for 3-4 minutes to let flavors meld.
5. Remove from heat, stir in sweetener if using.
6. Pour into mugs, sprinkle with extra cinnamon if desired.

For frothy version: Blend in a blender for 10 seconds before serving.

THE SCIENCE Curcumin reduces inflammatory markers (helpful for arthritis). Black pepper's piperine increases curcumin bioavailability by 2,000%. Ginger has anti-nausea and anti-inflammatory properties. Healthy fats (coconut oil) improve curcumin absorption.

NUTRITIONAL HIGHLIGHTS ~80 calories per serving | Rich in: Curcumin, Gingerol, Healthy fats

VARIATIONS

- Iced version: Blend all ingredients with ice
- Protein boost: Add protein powder
- Creamier: Use coconut milk
- Caffeine-free coffee substitute: Add ½ teaspoon instant coffee

STORAGE Best fresh. Can refrigerate up to 2 days; reheat gently or serve cold.

Recipe 24: Berry Brain Boost Smoothie

Memory • Focus • Antioxidants

SERVES: 2 | **PREP:** 5 min | **COOK:** 0 min

WHY IT WORKS *Blueberries protect neurons and improve memory. Spinach provides folate (brain health). Flax and walnuts add omega-3s. Green tea delivers L-theanine (calm focus). Perfect breakfast or pre-exam drink.*

INGREDIENTS

- 1 cup frozen blueberries
- ½ cup frozen strawberries
- 1 cup fresh spinach
- ½ frozen banana
- 2 tablespoons ground flaxseed
- 2 tablespoons chopped walnuts
- 1 cup cooled green tea (or water)
- ½ cup plain kefir or Greek yogurt
- Optional: 1 teaspoon honey

METHOD

1. Add all ingredients to a high-speed blender.
2. Blend on high for 60-90 seconds until completely smooth.
3. Add more liquid if too thick.
4. Pour into glasses and serve at once.

THE SCIENCE Blueberries' anthocyanins improve memory and protect against cognitive decline (Nutrients, 2020). Walnuts and flax provide omega-3s (brain structure and function). Spinach delivers folate (neurotransmitter synthesis). Green tea's L-theanine promotes calm alertness.

NUTRITIONAL HIGHLIGHTS ~260 calories per serving | Rich in: Antioxidants, Omega-3s (3g), Fiber (8g), Folate

VARIATIONS

- Extra protein: Add protein powder or extra yogurt
- Different berries: Try blackberries or raspberries
- Creamier: Add ¼ avocado
- Tropical: Replace berries with mango and pineapple

STORAGE Best fresh. Can refrigerate up to 24 hours; shake before drinking.

Recipe 25: Bone Broth (Regenerative)

Gut healing • Joint support • Immune recovery

SERVES: 8-10 cups | **PREP:** 15 min | **COOK:** 12-24 hours

WHY IT WORKS *Slow-simmered bones release collagen (which breaks down into gelatin), glycine and proline—amino acids that support tissue repair, gut lining integrity, and joint health. The addition of turmeric and ginger provides powerful anti-inflammatory compounds, while black pepper improves the absorption of curcumin from turmeric. This broth is ideal for recovery after illness, fasting, or physical stress.*

INGREDIENTS

For the broth:

- 2–3 lbs bones (chicken, beef, or fish bones)
- 2 tablespoons apple cider vinegar (helps extract minerals)
- 1 onion, quartered
- 3 carrots, chopped
- 3 celery stalks, chopped
- 4 garlic cloves, smashed
- 2–3 inch piece fresh ginger, sliced
- 1–2 inch piece fresh turmeric root, sliced (or 1 tsp turmeric powder)
- 1 tablespoon black peppercorns
- 2 bay leaves
- Fresh herbs (parsley, thyme, or rosemary)
- 12–16 cups water

To finish:

- Salt to taste
- Fresh lemon juice
- Optional: drizzle of extra-virgin olive oil

METHOD

Stovetop (12-24 hours):

1. Place bones in a large pot. Add vinegar and let sit for 30 minutes (extracts minerals).
2. Add onion, carrots, celery, garlic, ginger, turmeric, peppercorns, herbs, and water.
3. Bring to a boil, then reduce to the lowest simmer.
4. Cook for 12-24 hours (chicken: 12-18 hours; beef: 18-24 hours), skimming foam occasionally.
5. Strain through fine-mesh sieve.
6. Season with salt and lemon juice.

Instant Pot (3-4 hours):

1. Place all ingredients in Instant Pot.
2. Cook on high pressure for 3-4 hours.
3. Natural release, then strain.

Slow Cooker (12-24 hours):

1. Place all ingredients in slow cooker.
2. Cook on low for 12-24 hours.
3. Strain and season.

THE SCIENCE Bone broth provides collagen peptides, glycine (which supports gut lining repair, Nutrients, 2019), and proline (important for connective tissue). Turmeric contains curcumin, a compound studied for its anti-inflammatory and antioxidant effects. Ginger supports digestion and may help reduce inflammation and nausea. Together these ingredients create a nutrient-dense broth ideal for recovery and long-term health.

NUTRITIONAL HIGHLIGHTS ~40 calories per cup | Rich in: Collagen peptides, Glycine, Proline, Minerals (calcium, magnesium, phosphorus), anti-inflammatory polyphenols.

VARIATIONS

- Mediterranean herb broth: Add rosemary, thyme, garlic, and lemon peel during simmering. Finish with olive oil and fresh parsley.
- Mineral-rich broth: Add a strip of kombu (seaweed) during the final hour of cooking for additional trace minerals.
- Roasted bone broth: Roast bones at 400°F (200°C) for 30–40 minutes before simmering to deepen flavor and color.

STORAGE Refrigerate up to 5 days (fat will solidify on top—remove or leave for cooking fat). Freezes beautifully for 6 months in portions.

Recipe 26: Calming Chamomile-Lavender Tea

Sleep • Anxiety • Relaxation

SERVES: 2 | **PREP:** 2 min | **STEEP:** 7 min

WHY IT WORKS *Chamomile holds apigenin (binds to GABA receptors, promotes sleep). Lavender reduces anxiety and promotes relaxation. Lemon balm calms nervous system. Perfect bedtime ritual.*

INGREDIENTS

- 2 chamomile tea bags (or 2 tablespoons dried chamomile)
- 1 teaspoon dried culinary lavender
- 1 teaspoon dried lemon balm (optional)
- 2 cups boiling water
- 1 teaspoon honey (optional)
- Lemon slice (optional)

METHOD

1. Place chamomile, lavender, and lemon balm in a tea infuser or teapot.
2. Pour boiling water over herbs.
3. Cover and steep for 5-7 minutes.
4. Strain into cups.
5. Add honey and lemon if desired.
6. Sip slowly 30-60 minutes before bed.

THE SCIENCE Chamomile's apigenin binds to benzodiazepine receptors in the brain, promoting relaxation (Molecular Medicine Reports, 2010). Lavender reduces anxiety and improves sleep quality. Lemon balm has calming GABA-ergic effects.

NUTRITIONAL HIGHLIGHTS ~5 calories per serving | Rich in: Apigenin, Calming volatile oils

VARIATIONS

- Sleepy time blend: Add valerian root (strong sedative effect)
- Digestive: Add fresh ginger
- Iced version: Steep, chill, serve over ice with fresh mint

STORAGE Brew fresh each evening for best flavor and potency.

CLOSING: YOUR KITCHEN, YOUR PHARMACY

These 26 recipes stand for more than meals—they represent a complete approach to food as medicine. From breakfast to beverages, from quick snacks to healing dinners, each recipe is designed with specific health outcomes in mind. Your kitchen is now your pharmacy. Your recipes are now your prescriptions.

Cook with intention. Eat with gratitude. Heal with every bite.

References

Introduction & General

American Heart Association. (2022). Prevention and treatment of heart disease. Circulation, 145(8), e876-e894.

Centers for Disease Control and Prevention. (2022). Chronic disease prevention and health promotion. Atlanta, GA: CDC.

GBD 2017 Diet Collaborators. (2019). Health effects of dietary risks in 195 countries, 1990-2017: A systematic analysis for the Global Burden of Disease Study 2017. The Lancet, 393(10184), 1958-1972.

World Health Organization. (2022). Cardiovascular diseases fact sheet. Geneva: WHO.

Chapter 1: Food as the First Prescription

Mediterranean Diet Research:

Estruch, R., et al. (2013). Primary prevention of cardiovascular disease with a Mediterranean diet. New England Journal of Medicine, 368(14), 1279-1290.

Salas-Salvadó, J., et al. (2019). Effect of a lifestyle intervention program with energy-restricted Mediterranean diet and exercise on weight loss and cardiovascular risk factors. JAMA, 322(23), 2297-2309.

Blue Zones:

Buettner, D., & Skemp, S. (2016). Blue Zones: Lessons from the worlds longest lived. American Journal of Lifestyle Medicine, 10(5), 318-321.

Fiber and Health:

Reynolds, A., et al. (2019). Carbohydrate quality and human health: A series of systematic reviews and meta-analyses. The Lancet, 393(10170), 434-445.

Psychiatry and Nutrition:

Jacka, F. N., et al. (2017). A randomised controlled trial of dietary improvement for adults with major depression (the SMILES trial). BMC Medicine, 15(1), 23.

O'Neil, A., et al. (2014). Relationship between diet and mental health in children and adolescents. American Journal of Public Health, 104(10), e31-e42.

Chapter 2: Prevention Before Prescription

Cardiovascular Disease:

Mozaffarian, D., et al. (2020). Dietary olive oil and cardiovascular disease.

Journal of the American College of Cardiology, 75(15), 1729-1739.

Ornish, D., et al. (1990). Can lifestyle changes reverse coronary heart disease? JAMA, 263(21), 3007-3012.

Diabetes Prevention:

Diabetes Prevention Program Research Group. (2002). Reduction in the incidence of type 2 diabetes with lifestyle intervention or metformin. New England Journal of Medicine, 346(6), 393-403.

Satija, A., et al. (2016). Plant-based dietary patterns and incidence of type 2 diabetes. PLOS Medicine, 13(6), e1002039.

Cancer Prevention:

Clinton, S. K., et al. (2020). The World Cancer Research Fund/American Institute for Cancer Research third expert report on diet, nutrition, physical activity, and cancer. Cancer Research, 80(18), 3913-3927.

Song, M., et al. (2018). Association of animal and plant protein intake with all-cause and cause-specific mortality. JAMA Internal Medicine, 176(10), 1453-1463.

World Cancer Research Fund/American Institute for Cancer Research. (2018). Diet, nutrition, physical activity, and cancer: A global perspective. London: WCRF International.

DASH Diet:

Appel, L. J., et al. (1997). A clinical trial of the effects of dietary patterns on blood pressure. New England Journal of Medicine, 336(16), 1117-1124.

Sacks, F. M., et al. (2001). Effects on blood pressure of reduced dietary sodium and the Dietary Approaches to Stop Hypertension (DASH) diet. New England Journal of Medicine, 344(1), 3-10.

Chapter 3: Healing Chronic Illness & Mental Health

Depression and Diet:

Firth, J., et al. (2019). Food and mood: How do diet and nutrition affect mental wellbeing? BMJ, 369, m2382.

Lassale, C., et al. (2019). Healthy dietary indices and risk of depressive out-comes. Molecular Psychiatry, 24(7), 965-986.

Anxiety:

Aucoin, M., et al. (2021). Dietary interventions for anxiety. Frontiers in Psychiatry, 12, 663910.

Marx, W., et al. (2017). Diet and depression: Exploring the biological mechanisms. Molecular Psychiatry, 22(10), 1376-1387.

ADHD:

Chang, J. P., et al. (2018). Omega-3 polyunsaturated fatty acids in ADHD: A meta-analysis of randomized controlled trials. Journal of Clinical Psychiatry, 79(1), 16r11418.

Nigg, J. T., et al. (2017). Meta-analysis of attention-deficit/hyperactivity disorder and dietary nutrients. European Neuropsychopharmacology, 27(4), 331-343.

Bipolar Disorder:

Sarris, J., et al. (2016). Nutritional medicine as mainstream in psychiatry. Lancet Psychiatry, 2(3), 271-274.

Stoll, A. L., et al. (1999). Omega-3 fatty acids in bipolar disorder: A preliminary double-blind, placebo-controlled trial. Archives of General Psychiatry, 56(5), 407-412.

Trauma and PTSD:

Lopresti, A. L., et al. (2019). A review of lifestyle factors that contribute to mental health and well-being. Frontiers in Psychology, 10, 2016.

Vujanovic, A. A., et al. (2020). Exercise and PTSD symptoms. Journal of Psychiatric Research, 129, 194-201.

Cancer and Nutrition:

Farvid, M. S., et al. (2018). Fruit and vegetable consumption and breast cancer incidence. International Journal of Cancer, 142(10), 1968-1980.

Rock, C. L., et al. (2020). American Cancer Society guideline for diet and physical activity for cancer prevention. CA: A Cancer Journal for Clini-cians, 70(4), 245-271.

Gut-Brain Axis:

Cryan, J. F., et al. (2019). The microbiota-gut-brain axis. Physiological Reviews, 99(4), 1877-2013.

Chapter 4: The Science of Longevity

Telomeres:

Ornish, D., et al. (2008). Increased telomerase activity and comprehensive lifestyle changes. The Lancet Oncology, 9(11), 1048-1057.

Ornish, D., et al. (2013). Effect of comprehensive lifestyle changes on telomerase activity and telomere length in men with low-risk prostate cancer. The Lancet Oncology, 14(11), 1112-1120.

Mitochondria:

López-Lluch, G., et al. (2018). Mitochondrial biogenesis and healthy aging. Experimental Gerontology, 56, 116-127.

Sánchez-Román, I., et al. (2011). Forty percent methionine restriction lowers DNA methylation, complex I ROS generation, and oxidative damage to mtDNA and mitochondrial proteins in rat heart. Journal of Bioenergetics and Biomembranes, 43(6), 699-708.

NAD+ and Aging:

Yoshino, J., et al. (2018). NAD+ intermediates: The biology and therapeutic potential of NMN and NR. Cell Metabolism, 27(3), 513-528.

Zhang, H., et al. (2016). NAD+ repletion improves mitochondrial and stem cell function and enhances life span in mice. Science, 352(6292), 1436-1443.

Fasting:

de Cabo, R., & Mattson, M. P. (2019). Effects of intermittent fasting on health, aging, and disease. New England Journal of Medicine, 381(26), 2541-2551.

Longo, V. D., & Mattson, M. P. (2014). Fasting: Molecular mechanisms and clinical applications. Cell Metabolism, 19(2), 181-192.

Stem Cells and Nutrition:

Cheng, C. W., et al. (2014). Prolonged fasting reduces IGF-1/PKA to pro-mote hematopoietic-stem-cell-based regeneration and reverse immunosuppression. Cell Stem Cell, 14(6), 810-823.

Precision Nutrition:

Zeevi, D., et al. (2015). Personalized nutrition by prediction of glycemic responses. Cell, 163(5), 1079-1094.

Microbiome:

Claesson, M. J., et al. (2012). Gut microbiota composition correlates with diet and health in the elderly. Nature, 488(7410), 178-184.

Mariat, D., et al. (2009). The Firmicutes/Bacteroidetes ratio of the human microbiota changes with age. BMC Microbiology, 9(1), 123.

Blue Zones:

Buettner, D. (2012). The Blue Zones: 9 lessons for living longer from the people who have lived the longest. National Geographic Books.

Willcox, D. C., et al. (2014). Healthy aging diets other than the Mediterranean. Mechanisms of Ageing and Development, 136-137, 148-162.

Chapter 5: Peak Performance

Exercise and Mental Health:

Schuch, F. B., et al. (2018). Exercise as a treatment for depression: A meta-analysis adjusting for publication bias. Journal of Psychiatric Research, 77, 42-51.

Stubbs, B., et al. (2017). An examination of the anxiolytic effects of exercise for people with anxiety and stress-related disorders. Psychiatry Research, 249, 102-108.

Sports Nutrition:

Jäger, R., et al. (2017). International Society of Sports Nutrition position stand: Protein and exercise. Journal of the International Society of Sports Nutrition, 14(1), 20.

Thomas, D. T., et al. (2016). American College of Sports Medicine joint position statement: Nutrition and athletic performance. Medicine & Science in Sports & Exercise, 48(3), 543-568.

ADHD and Exercise:

Den Heijer, A. E., et al. (2017). Sweat it out? The effects of physical exercise on cognition and behavior in children and adults with ADHD. Journal of Neural Transmission, 124(1), 3-26.

Recovery and Regenerative Medicine:

Andia, I., & Maffulli, N. (2013). Platelet-rich plasma for managing pain and inflammation in osteoarthritis. Nature Reviews Rheumatology, 9(12), 721-730.

Centeno, C. J., et al. (2018). A specific protocol of autologous bone marrow concentrates and platelet products versus exercise therapy. International Orthopaedics, 42(9), 2127-2134.

Chapter 6: The Roadmap to Regeneration

Lifestyle Medicine:

Freeman, A. M., et al. (2017). Trending cardiovascular nutrition controversies. Journal of the American College of Cardiology, 69(9), 1172-1187.

Katz, D. L., & Meller, S. (2014). Can we say what diet is best for health?

Annual Review of Public Health, 35, 83-103.

Economics of Prevention:

Barnard, N. D., et al. (2009). A low-fat vegan diet and a conventional diabetes diet in the treatment of type 2 diabetes. American Journal of Clinical Nutrition, 89(5), 1588S-1596S.

Tuso, P. J., et al. (2013). Nutritional update for physicians: Plant-based diets. Permanente Journal, 17(2), 61-66.

Behavioral Change:

Gardner, B., et al. (2012). Making health habitual: The psychology of 'habit-formation' and general practice. British Journal of General Practice, 62(605), 664-666.

Lally, P., et al. (2010). How are habits formed: Modelling habit formation in the real world. European Journal of Social Psychology, 40(6), 998-1009.

Chapter 7: Recipes for Life

Cooking and Nutrient Retention:

Miglio, C., et al. (2008). Effects of different cooking methods on nutritional and physicochemical characteristics of selected vegetables. Journal of Agricultural and Food Chemistry, 56(1), 139-147.

Olive Oil:

Schwingshackl, L., et al. (2014). Monounsaturated fatty acids and risk of cardiovascular disease. Circulation Research, 124(10), 1341-1354.

Turmeric and Curcumin:

Hewlings, S. J., & Kalman, D. S. (2017). Curcumin: A review of its effects on human health. Foods, 6(10), 92.

Shoba, G., et al. (1998). Influence of piperine on the pharmacokinetics of curcumin in animals and human volunteers. Planta Medica, 64(4), 353-356.

Omega-3 Fatty Acids:

Calder, P. C. (2017). Omega-3 fatty acids and inflammatory processes. Nutrients, 9(11), 1273.

Mozaffarian, D., & Wu, J. H. (2011). Omega-3 fatty acids and cardiovascular disease. Journal of the American College of Cardiology, 58(20), 2047-2067.

Appendix A: Shopping Lists & Pantry Essentials

The Foundation Pantry

Legumes (Dried & Canned):

- Brown lentils
- Red lentils
- Green lentils
- Chickpeas (garbanzo beans)
- Black beans
- White beans (cannellini, navy)
- Kidney beans
- Pinto beans

Whole Grains:

- Rolled oats (old-fashioned)
- Steel-cut oats
- Quinoa (white, red, or tricolor)
- Brown rice
- Barley (pearl or hulled)
- Bulgur

- Farro
- Whole grain pasta
- Whole grain bread (sourdough preferred)

Nuts & Seeds:

- Walnuts
- Almonds
- Cashews
- Pecans
- Chia seeds
- Ground flaxseed
- Pumpkin seeds (pepitas)
- Sunflower seeds
- Hemp seeds
- Sesame seeds
- Tahini (sesame seed paste)

Oils & Fats:

- Extra virgin olive oil (primary cooking oil)
- Avocado oil (high-heat cooking)
- Coconut oil (occasional use)
- Sesame oil (flavoring)

Canned/Jarred Goods:

- Crushed tomatoes
- Diced tomatoes
- Tomato paste
- Vegetable broth (low sodium)

- Sardines (in water or olive oil)
- Wild-caught salmon (canned)
- Olives (Kalamata, green)
- Capers

Spices & Herbs:

- Turmeric powder
- Cumin (ground)
- Coriander (ground)
- Paprika (regular and smoked)
- Cinnamon
- Ginger powder
- Garlic powder
- Onion powder
- Oregano (dried)
- Basil (dried)
- Thyme (dried)
- Rosemary (dried)
- Bay leaves
- Black pepper (whole peppercorns + grinder)
- Sea salt or Himalayan pink salt
- Red pepper flakes

Vinegars & Condiments:

- Apple cider vinegar
- Balsamic vinegar
- Red wine vinegar

- Low-sodium soy sauce or tamari
- Dijon mustard
- Miso paste (white or red)
- Nutritional yeast (for "cheesy" flavor)

Sweeteners (Use Sparingly):

- Raw honey
- Pure maple syrup
- Medjool dates

Weekly Fresh List

Proteins:

- Wild-caught salmon (fresh or frozen)
- Sardines (fresh if available)
- Eggs (pasture-raised preferred)
- Plain Greek yogurt or kefir
- Organic chicken (if consuming meat)
- Tofu or tempeh

Vegetables (Prioritize Variety):

- Leafy greens: Spinach, kale, arugula, Swiss chard, collard greens
- Cruciferous: Broccoli, cauliflower, Brussels sprouts, cabbage
- Alliums: Onions, garlic, shallots, leeks
- Nightshades: Tomatoes, bell peppers (all colors), eggplant
- Root vegetables: Carrots, sweet potatoes, beets, radishes
- Others: Zucchini, cucumber, celery, mushrooms, asparagus

Fruits:

- Berries: Blueberries, strawberries, raspberries, blackberries (fresh or frozen)

- Citrus: Lemons, limes, oranges, grapefruit
- Other: Apples, bananas, pomegranates, avocados
- Frozen: Mixed berries (for smoothies)

Fresh Herbs:

- Parsley
- Cilantro
- Basil
- Mint
- Rosemary
- Thyme

Budget-Friendly Shopping Tips

- Buy in bulk: Beans, grains, nuts, and seeds are cheaper in bulk bins
- Choose frozen: Frozen vegetables and berries are just as nutritious and often cheaper
- Seasonal produce: Buy fruits and vegetables in season for better prices
- Store brands: Generic/store brands are often identical quality at lower cost
- Canned is fine: Canned beans and tomatoes are budget-friendly and nutritious
- Skip "superfoods": Regular vegetables work just as well as expensive trendy items
- Meal prep: Cooking at home is always cheaper than eating out
- Grow herbs: Fresh herbs are expensive to buy but easy to grow on a windowsill

Storage Tips

Pantry Items:

- Store nuts and seeds in airtight containers in refrigerator or freezer (prevents rancidity)
- Keep grains in sealed containers to prevent pests
- Olive oil should be stored in dark, cool place (not above stove)

Produce:

- Store leafy greens in breathable produce bags in refrigerator
- Keep tomatoes at room temperature for best flavor
- Store onions and garlic in cool, dark, dry place (not refrigerator)
- Berries: Wash only when ready to use; store in refrigerator

Batch Cooking:

- Cooked beans: Refrigerate up to 5 days, freeze up to 6 months
- Cooked grains: Refrigerate up to 5 days, freeze up to 3 months
- Roasted vegetables: Refrigerate up to 5 days
- Soups and stews: Refrigerate up to 5 days, freeze up to 3 months

Appendix B: Meal Planning Templates

Template 1: Weekly Meal Prep Planner

Sunday Prep Session (90 minutes):

Grains (Choose 2):

- Cook quinoa (3 cups)
- Cook brown rice (3 cups)
- Cook barley (2 cups)

Proteins (Choose 2-3):

- Cook beans/lentils (2 pots)
- Boil eggs (6-12)
- Bake salmon or chicken
- Prep tofu/tempeh

Vegetables:

- Roast 2 sheet pans of vegetables
- Wash and chop salad greens
- Prep raw snack vegetables

Other:

- Make salad dressing (lemon-olive oil)
- Portion nuts/seeds into snack bags
- Cut fruit for the week

Template 2: Daily Meal Structure

Breakfast (Choose one):

- Overnight oats with berries and walnuts
- Greek yogurt with nuts and fruit
- Eggs with vegetables and whole grain toast
- Smoothie with greens, berries, protein
- Chia pudding

Lunch (Choose one):

- Grain bowl (grain + beans + vegetables + dressing)
- Soup + whole grain bread
- Salad with protein
- Leftovers from dinner
- Wrap or sandwich

Dinner (Template):

- Protein (palm-sized part)
- Vegetables (half the plate)
- Whole grain or starchy vegetable (quarter of plate)
- Healthy fat (olive oil, avocado, nuts)

Snacks (Choose 1-2):

- Fruit + nuts
- Hummus + vegetables
- Energy balls

- Roasted chickpeas
- Apple with almond butter

Template 3: 7-Day Mix-and-Match Planner

Proteins (Choose 7 for the week):

1. Turmeric lentil soup
2. Black beans
3. Chickpeas
4. Salmon
5. Sardines
6. Eggs
7. Greek yogurt/kefir

Vegetables (Aim for 7-9 servings daily):

- Leafy greens (spinach, kale, arugula)
- Cruciferous (broccoli, Brussels sprouts)
- Colorful (peppers, tomatoes, carrots)
- Alliums (onions, garlic)

Grains (Choose 3-4 for the week):

1. Quinoa
2. Brown rice
3. Oats
4. Barley
5. Whole grain bread

Healthy Fats (Daily):

- Olive oil (3-4 tablespoons)
- Nuts/seeds (¼ cup)

- Avocado (½)

Template 4: Grocery List Generator

Proteins:

- Beans/lentils: ______________________________
- Fish: ______________________________
- Eggs: ______________________________
- Yogurt/kefir: ______________________________

Grains:

- Breakfast grain: ______________________________
- Lunch/dinner grain: ______________________________
- Bread: ______________________________

Vegetables (Aim for 15+ items):

- Leafy greens: ______________________________
- Cruciferous: ______________________________
- Nightshades: ______________________________
- Root vegetables: ______________________________
- Alliums: ______________________________
- Others: ______________________________

Fruits:

- Berries: ______________________________
- Citrus: ______________________________
- Other: ______________________________

Fats:

- Olive oil: ______________________________
- Nuts: ______________________________

- Seeds: ____________________
- Avocados ____________________

Pantry Restocks:

- ____________________
- ____________________

Appendix C: Recommended Resources

Books

Nutrition Science:

- How Not to Die by Michael Greger, MD
- The Blue Zones by Dan Buettner
- In Defense of Food by Michael Pollan
- Food Rules by Michael Pollan
- The China Study by T. Colin Campbell

Nutritional Psychiatry:

- The Food-Mood Connection by Uma Naidoo, MD
- This is Your Brain on Food by Uma Naidoo, MD
- The Happiness Diet by Tyler G. Graham and Drew Ramsey, MD

Longevity and Anti-Aging:

- Lifespan by David Sinclair, PhD
- The Longevity Diet by Valter Longo, PhD
- Life Force by Tony Robbins, Peter Diamandis, and Robert Hariri

Cookbooks:

- The Mediterranean Diet Cookbook by Martina Slajerova
- How to Cook Everything Vegetarian by Mark Bittman
- Plenty by Yotam Ottolenghi

Websites & Apps

Nutrition Information:

- NutritionFacts.org (Dr. Michael Greger's clinically proven nutrition)
- Examine.com (supplement research)
- PubMed.gov (scientific research database)

Meal Planning:

- PlantYou (plant-based meal planning)
- Paprika App (recipe management and meal planning)
- Mealime (healthy meal planning)

Food Tracking (if helpful for you):

- Cronometer (nutrient tracking)
- MyFitnessPal (food diary)

Shopping:

- Thrive Market (healthy groceries delivered)
- Imperfect Foods (reduce food waste, save money)

Professional Organizations

Find Registered Dietitians:

- Academy of Nutrition and Dietetics (eatright.org)
- American College of Lifestyle Medicine (lifestylemedicine.org)
- Plantrician Project (plant-based nutrition experts)

Mental Health:

- American Psychiatric Association (psychiatry.org)
- Anxiety and Depression Association of America (adaa.org)
- National Alliance on Mental Illness (nami.org)

Integrative and Functional Medicine:

- Institute for Functional Medicine (ifm.org)
- American Board of Integrative Medicine (abim.org)

Podcasts

- The Rich Roll Podcast (health, fitness, nutrition)
- Found My Fitness with Dr. Rhonda Patrick (longevity science)
- The Model Health Show with Shawn Stevenson
- The Food Psych Podcast with Christy Harrison

Lab Testing (Discuss with your physician)

Basic Health Markers:

- Complete metabolic panel
- Lipid panel (cholesterol, triglycerides)
- HbA1c (blood sugar control)
- Complete blood count
- Thyroid panel (TSH, T3, T4)
- Vitamin D levels
- Vitamin B12 levels

Advanced (Optional):

- Omega-3 index
- hs-CRP (inflammation marker)
- Homocysteine

- Microbiome testing
- Continuous glucose monitor (CGM)

Support & Community

Online Communities:

- r/PlantBasedDiet (Reddit)
- r/EatCheapAndHealthy (Reddit)
- Blue Zones Project communities
- Local cooking classes and meal prep groups

Accountability:

- Find a cooking friend
- Join a walking group
- Hire a health coach or nutritionist
- Work with a therapist for emotional eating support

Acknowledgments

This book would not exist without the countless patients who trusted me with their stories, their struggles, and their triumphs. You taught me that healing is not a one-way street—it is a shared journey. Your courage to change inspired every page.

To my husband, who resisted healthy eating for years until a blood pressure reading changed everything. Your transformation from skeptic to believer reminded me that it is never too late to choose health. Thank you for letting me share your story.

To my colleagues in psychiatry, integrative medicine, and nutrition science, who bridge the worlds of rigorous research and compassionate care. Your work proves that food is not "alternative" medicine—it is foundational medicine.

To my family, whose health stories—both the struggles and the victories—shaped my understanding of prevention, resilience, and the excessive cost of ignoring lifestyle medicine.

To the researchers whose studies fill the references section of this book: your dedication to scientific truth gives patients hope and physicians evidence.

To my teachers in Brazil and the United States, who taught me to think critically, to question assumptions, and to never stop learning.

To the Blue Zones communities—Okinawa, Sardinia, Ikaria, Nicoya, and Loma Linda—whose centenarians showed us that longevity is not genetics alone, but daily choices compounded over decades.

To every reader who picks up this book: you deserve to know that your health is not predetermined. You have more power than you realize. The food on your plate shapes your future.

And finally, to those struggling with ADHD, depression, anxiety, trauma, chronic illness, or simply the challenge of showing up for yourself every day: I see you. I have been there. If my journey from fourteen-year-old giving up sugar to physician fighting through ADHD to pass my final licensing exam proves anything, it is this: change is possible. Healing is possible. And you do not have to do it alone.

Thank you for trusting me with your time and your health. May this book be the beginning of your transformation.

With gratitude and hope, Dr. Daniela T. Rizzo, M.D.

A Final Note from the Author

If you take only one message from this book, let it be this: You are not powerless.

You can lower your risk of heart disease by 30%. You can cut your risk of diabetes in half.

You can triple your chance of depression remission.

You can protect your brain, strengthen your bones, brighten your skin, and extend your years—not with a miracle drug, but with what you put on your plate.

The science is clear. The stories are real. The choice is yours.

I gave up sugar at fourteen because I refused to accept my family's fate.

I fought through ADHD because I believed food and focus could work together.

I watched my husband reverse hypertension in three months because he finally chose change.

I have seen patients overcome diabetes, depression, cancer recurrence, and trauma—one meal, one day, one choice at a time.

If we can do it, so can you. Your kitchen is your pharmacy.

Your recipes are your prescriptions.

Your future begins now—on your plate, in your body, through your choices.

Welcome to regeneration.
With hope and conviction,
Dr. Daniela T. Rizzo, M.D.

www.ingramcontent.com/pod-product-compliance
Lightning Source LLC
LaVergne TN
LVHW081633120826
845149LV00025B/1887
9798995417910